PROFESSIONAL ISSUES FOR TODAY'S NURSE

PROFESSIONAL ISSUES FOR TODAY'S NURSE

Allison J. Terry
WALDEN UNIVERSITY

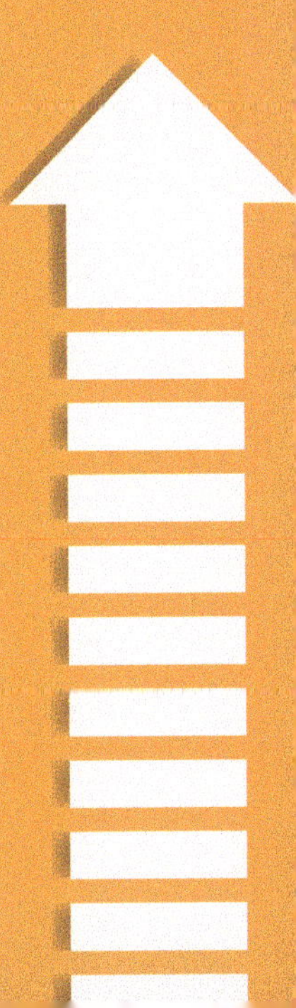

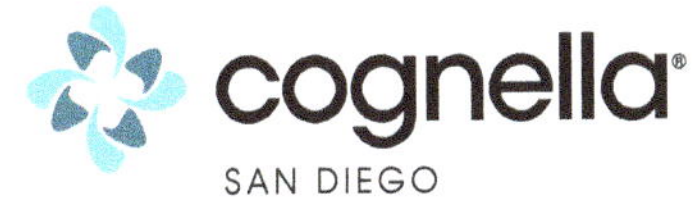

Bassim Hamadeh, CEO and Publisher
Amanda Martin, Publisher
Amy Smith, Senior Project Editor
Alia Bales, Production Manager
Emely Villavicencio, Senior Graphic Designer
Kylie Bartolome, Licensing Specialist
Natalie Piccotti, Director of Marketing
Kassie Graves, Senior Vice Presiden, Editorial
Jamie Giganti, Director of Academic Publishing

Printed in the United States of America

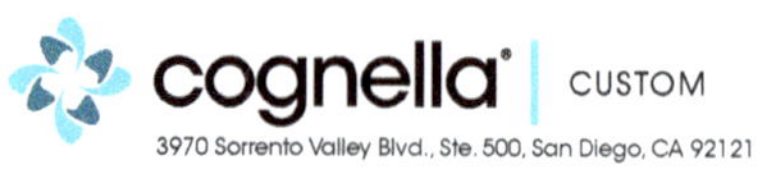

This book is dedicated to my husband and my parents.

Brief Contents

Preface xv

PART 1 **Development of Nursing as a Profession** 1

CHAPTER 1 History of Nursing as a Profession 2
CHAPTER 2 Nursing Theory 31
CHAPTER 3 Nursing Licensure 75

PART 2 **Transition Into the Professional Nurse Role** 91

CHAPTER 4 Ethical Issues in Nursing 92
CHAPTER 5 Legal Aspects of Nursing 110
CHAPTER 6 Cultural Aspects of Nursing 131
CHAPTER 7 Informatics 152
CHAPTER 8 Teaching-Learning Process 167
CHAPTER 9 The Nursing Process 182
CHAPTER 10 Spirituality 212

PART 3 **Nursing Leadership and Management** 223

CHAPTER 11 Communication as a Registered Nurse 224
CHAPTER 12 Delegation 251
CHAPTER 13 Conflict Management 261
CHAPTER 14 Supervision 273
CHAPTER 15 Quality Improvement 286
CHAPTER 16 Health Care Delivery Systems 298

PART 4 **Current Issues in Health Care Delivery** 313

CHAPTER 17 Disaster Preparedness 314
CHAPTER 18 Nursing Workforce Shortage 328
CHAPTER 19 Violence in the Workplace 341

Index 353

Detailed Contents

Preface . . . xv

PART 1 **Development of Nursing as a Profession** 1

CHAPTER 1 **History of Nursing as a Profession** . . . 2

Origins of Nursing . . . 2
Transition to Secular Nursing . . . 4
Emergence of Modern Nursing . . . 6
Nursing During the Civil War . . . 7
Development of Schools of Nursing . . . 10
Nursing During World War I . . . 11
Nursing During World War II . . . 12
Nursing During the Vietnam War . . . 13
Twenty-First Century Nursing . . . 14
Role Evolution in Modern Nursing . . . 14
Summary of Key Points in Chapter . . . 15
Conclusion . . . 16
Critical Thinking Questions . . . 18
Scenarios . . . 20
NCLEX-Style Review Questions . . . 22
Note Taker . . . 25
References . . . 29

CHAPTER 2 **Nursing Theory** . . . 31

Introduction to Nursing Theory . . . 31
- Florence Nightingale's Theory of Nursing . . . 32
- Hildegard Peplau's Theory of Nursing . . . 34
- Virginia Henderson's Theory of Nursing . . . 35
- Ida Orlando's Theory of Nursing . . . 37
- Martha Rogers' Theory of Nursing . . . 39
- Sister Callista Roy's Theory of Nursing . . . 41
- Imogene King's Theory of Nursing . . . 42
- Dorothea Orem's Theory of Nursing . . . 44
- Betty Neuman's Theory of Nursing . . . 46
- Jean Watson's Theory of Human Science and Human Caring . . . 47

Summary of Key Points in Chapter 49
Conclusion 50
Critical Thinking Questions 50
Scenarios 58
NCLEX-Style Review Questions 66
Note Taker 68
References 74

CHAPTER 3 **Nursing Licensure** 75
Introduction to the Nursing Licensure Process 75
Sustaining Discipline of a Nursing License 77
Summary of Key Points in Chapter 79
Conclusion 79
Critical Thinking Questions 80
Scenarios 81
NCLEX-Style Review Questions 83
Case Study 84
Concept Map 85
Note Taker 85
References 90

PART 2 **Transition Into the Professional Nurse Role** **91**

CHAPTER 4 **Ethical Issues in Nursing** 92
ANA Code of Ethics 93
Ethical Decision-Making 93
Ethical Issues Related to Death and Dying 94
Moral Distress 95
Summary of Key Points in Chapter 96
Conclusion 97
Critical Thinking Questions 97
Scenarios 100
NCLEX-Style Review Questions 101
Case Study 102
Concept Map 103
Notetaker 103
References 109

CHAPTER 5 **Legal Aspects of Nursing** 110
Public Law 110
Civil Law 112
Advanced Directives 113
  Informed Consent 113
Issues Involving Confidentiality 114
Summary of Key Points in Chapter 114
Conclusion 114
Critical Thinking Questions 115
Scenarios 118

NCLEX-Style Review Questions . . . 122
Case Study . . . 123
Concept Map . . . 124
Note Taker . . . 125
References . . . 130

CHAPTER 6 **Cultural Aspects of Nursing** . . . 131
Introduction . . . 131
Cultural Humility . . . 132
Overview of Culture . . . 133
Functioning as a Culture . . . 134
Vulnerable Populations . . . 135
Healthy People 2030 . . . 135
Need for Health Equity . . . 136
Summary of Key Points in Chapter . . . 138
Conclusion . . . 139
Critical Thinking Questions . . . 139
Scenarios . . . 143
NCLEX-Style Review Questions . . . 146
New Format NCLEX Questions . . . 147
Case Study . . . 148
Concept Map . . . 149
Note Taker . . . 149
References . . . 151

CHAPTER 7 **Informatics** . . . 152
Telehealth . . . 153
Electronic Health Records . . . 155
Summary of Key Points in Chapter . . . 157
Conclusion . . . 157
Critical Thinking Questions . . . 157
Scenarios . . . 159
NCLEX-Style Review Questions . . . 160
Case Study . . . 160
Concept Map . . . 162
Note Taker . . . 162
References . . . 166

CHAPTER 8 **Teaching-Learning Process** . . . 167
Steps in the Teaching-Learning Process . . . 167
How to Make Your Patient Teaching More Effective . . . 170
Summary of Key Points in Chapter . . . 171
Conclusion . . . 171
Critical Thinking Questions . . . 171
Scenarios . . . 173
NCLEX-Style Review Questions . . . 175
Case Study . . . 175
Concept Map . . . 176

Note Taker . . . 176
References . . . 181

CHAPTER 9 **The Nursing Process** . . . 182
Introduction to the Nursing Process . . . 182
Assessment . . . 183
Diagnosis . . . 185
Planning . . . 197
Intervention . . . 198
Evaluation . . . 200
Concept Mapping . . . 200
Summary of Key Points in Chapter . . . 201
Conclusion . . . 202
Critical Thinking Questions . . . 202
Scenarios . . . 204
NCLEX-Style Review Questions . . . 206
New Format NCLEX-Type Questions . . . 208
Case Study . . . 209
Concept Map . . . 209
Note Taker . . . 210
References . . . 211

CHAPTER 10 **Spirituality** . . . 212
Conducting a Spiritual Assessment . . . 212
Developing Knowledge and Skills to Assess Patients' Spiritual Needs . . . 214
Implementing Spiritual Nursing Care Behaviors in Clinical Practice . . . 214
Summary of Key Points in Chapter . . . 215
Conclusion . . . 215
Critical Thinking Questions . . . 215
Scenarios . . . 216
NCLEX-Style Review Questions . . . 217
Case Study . . . 218
Concept Map . . . 220
Note Taker . . . 220
References . . . 222

PART 3 **Nursing Leadership and Management** **223**

CHAPTER 11 **Communication as a Registered Nurse** . . . 224
Introduction to the Communication Process . . . 224
Process of Communication . . . 225
Modes and Channels of Communication . . . 226
Verbal Communication in Nursing . . . 227
Nonverbal Communication in Nursing . . . 229
Email . . . 229
Incongruent Communication . . . 230
Barriers to Communication . . . 231
Communication With Peers . . . 234

Communication With Subordinates . . . 235
Communication With Physicians . . . 236
Communicating With Upper-Level Management . . . 237
Summary of Key Points in Chapter . . . 238
Conclusion . . . 239
Critical Thinking Questions . . . 239
Scenarios . . . 241
NCLEX-Style Review Questions . . . 244
Case Study . . . 246
Concept Map . . . 247
Note Taker . . . 247
References . . . 249

CHAPTER 12 **Delegation** . . . 251
Barriers to Using Delegation Appropriately . . . 252
Delegating an Intervention to an Unlicensed Person . . . 252
Skills Needed to Set Priorities . . . 253
Summary of Key Points in Chapter . . . 254
Conclusion . . . 254
Critical Thinking Questions . . . 254
Scenarios . . . 255
NCLEX-Style Review Questions . . . 256
Case Study . . . 257
Concept Map . . . 258
Note Taker . . . 258
References . . . 260

CHAPTER 13 **Conflict Management** . . . 261
Stages of Conflict . . . 261
Types of Power . . . 262
Responses to Conflict . . . 263
Conflict Resolution . . . 263
Summary of Key Points in Chapter . . . 264
Conclusion . . . 264
Critical Thinking Questions . . . 265
Scenarios . . . 266
NCLEX-Style Review Questions . . . 267
Case Study . . . 268
Concept Map . . . 269
Note Taker . . . 269
References . . . 272

CHAPTER 14 **Supervision** . . . 273
Supervision . . . 273
Developing Effective Clinical Supervision . . . 274
Barriers to Effective Clinical Supervision . . . 274
Summary of Key Points in Chapter . . . 276
Conclusion . . . 276

Critical Thinking Questions ... 276
Scenarios ... 278
NCLEX-Style Review Questions ... 280
Case Study ... 280
Concept Map ... 281
Note Taker ... 281
References ... 285

CHAPTER 15 **Quality Improvement** ... 286
Performance Measurement ... 286
Sentinel Events ... 287
Summary of Key Points in Chapter ... 289
Conclusion ... 289
Critical Thinking Questions ... 289
Scenarios ... 291
NCLEX-Style Review Questions ... 293
Case Study ... 293
Concept Map ... 294
Note Taker ... 294
References ... 297

CHAPTER 16 **Health Care Delivery Systems** ... 298
Managed Care Organizations ... 298
Integrated Delivery System ... 299
Self-Directed Services ... 300
Telehealth ... 300
Summary of Key Points in Chapter ... 301
Conclusion ... 301
Critical Thinking Questions ... 301
Scenarios ... 303
NCLEX-Style Review Questions ... 305
Case Study ... 306
Concept Map ... 307
Note Taker ... 307
References ... 311

PART 4 Current Issues in Health Care Delivery 313

CHAPTER 17 **Disaster Preparedness** ... 314
Stages of Disaster Preparedness ... 315
Stages of Emergency Management ... 317
Summary of Key Points in Chapter ... 318
Conclusion ... 318
Critical Thinking Questions ... 318
Scenarios ... 320
NCLEX-Style Review Questions ... 322
Case Study ... 323
Concept Map ... 324

Note Taker . . . 324
References . . . 327

CHAPTER 18 **Nursing Workforce Shortage** . . . 328
Why Are Nurses Leaving Bedside Nursing? . . . 329
Improving the Current Nursing Shortage . . . 329
Summary of Key Points in Chapter . . . 331
Conclusion . . . 331
Critical Thinking Questions . . . 331
Scenarios . . . 333
NCLEX-Style Review Questions . . . 335
Case Study . . . 336
Concept Map . . . 337
Note Taker . . . 337
References . . . 340

CHAPTER 19 **Violence in the Workplace** . . . 341
Types of Workplace Violence . . . 341
Workplace Incivility . . . 342
Preventing Violence Against Health Care Workers . . . 342
Summary of Key Points in Chapter . . . 344
Conclusion . . . 344
Critical Thinking Questions . . . 344
Scenarios . . . 346
NCLEX-Style Review Questions . . . 348
Case Study . . . 349
Concept Map . . . 350
Note Taker . . . 350
References . . . 352

Index . . . **353**

Preface

Healthcare in general and nursing specifically were changed forever by the recent pandemic. As a result, emerging 21st-century nurse leaders will be faced with challenges never imagined by earlier generations. How can subsequent generations of nurses be prepared for these challenges? Whereas nurses once carried clipboards with important notes for their day of patient care, today's nurses must have a virtual toolbox at their disposal to cope with each obstacle to be encountered. This book hopes to add to the post-COVID 19 nurse's virtual toolbox. Pedagogical features included in the book that may prove to be useful include critical thinking questions, scenarios to generate class discussion, new-format NCLEX-type questions, note-taker documents to increase test preparation, and case studies to stimulate critical thinking and problem-solving skills.

As today's nurses help redefine the features of post-COVID 19 healthcare, some basic challenges remain unchanged: having sufficient problem solving and critical thinking skills along with NCLEX preparation to ensure that the nurse can enter the profession and smoothly transition into a practicing role. It is the author's hope that this book will facilitate that transition.

PART I

Development of Nursing as a Profession

CHAPTER

1

History of Nursing as a Profession

CHAPTER OBJECTIVES

Upon completion of the chapter, you will be able to:

1. Discuss the development of nursing as a profession from ancient times until the 19th century
2. Describe how Florence Nightingale came to be seen as the founder of modern nursing
3. Discuss the contributions of early nurses such as Dorothea Dix, Clara Barton, Linda Richards, and Mary Eliza Mahoney to the development of modern nursing
4. Discuss the contributions of nurses during wartime
5. Describe the roles of the doctor of nursing practice and clinical nurse leader in the modern health care community

KEY TERMS

advanced practice nurses
Annie G. Fox
Brahmanism
Clara Barton
clinical nurse leader
Colonel Anna May Hays
Colonel Mildred Clark
deaconess
Deborah
doctor of nursing practice
Dorothea Dix
Edith Nourse Rogers
Ednah Dow Cheney
Edwin Smith surgical papyrus
Florence Nightingale
Helen Fairchild
Kate Cumming
Linda Richards
Marie Zakrzewska
Mary Eliza Mahoney
Mosaic Law
New England Hospital for Women and Children
papyrus
Paula of Actin
Sally Louisa Tompkins
Theodor Fliedner
Thomas Fuller
Valentine Seaman
Vivien Bullwinkel
widow

Origins of Nursing

Nursing has been referred to as both the oldest art and the youngest profession. Its origins can be traced back to the dawn of civilization through the traditional mother-child relationship as well as to the important role of the village healer in many primitive societies. However, in more sophisticated societies, such as that of ancient Egypt, the importance of the nursing discipline became evident as nurses assisted in the recovery of patients experiencing traumatic injuries, such as those sustained on the battlefield.

A papyrus dating back to the 17th century B.C., known as the *Edwin Smith surgical papyrus*, is one of the oldest documents pertaining to medicine. It is the earliest known surgical prototype textbook and lists the proper surgical treatment for a variety of traumatic injuries that begin with the head and proceed downward anatomically. Although magic was considered a major part of medical treatment at the time, the Edwin Smith papyrus resorts to the use of magic in only one described case, relying instead on descriptions of the logical treatment of patients (Nunn, 2008).

The origins of many of the practices still used in modern nursing can be seen in the directives of the **Mosaic Law** that was followed by the ancient Israelites from the 15th century B.C. until the first century A.D., when the Jews began to be dispersed throughout the known world. As in many societies of that era, responsibility for the health of the public rested with the male-dominated priestly tribe of the Levites. The people were taught to prevent disease through a regimen of personal hygiene and specific times set aside for work, rest, and sleep. Specific and detailed instructions were provided regarding:

- The proper treatment of women during pregnancy, childbirth, and menstruation
- The selection of food that met dietary requirements
- Recognizing communicable disease so that priests could be notified of an outbreak
- When to implement quarantine procedures

The Bible has the distinction of being the document that records the first nurse mentioned by name in history. **Deborah** was recorded in the 24th chapter of the book of Genesis as being the nurse of Rebekah, who was traveling to meet her future husband, Isaac (Donahue, 2010).

Hygiene and the prevention of illness were further emphasized by Indian **Brahmanism** after 1500 B.C. The religion's teachings included topics such as medicine and surgery. Indian surgery was considered to be the most highly skilled of any of the known ancient civilizations.

Brahmanism, also referred to as *Hinduism*, further emphasized the importance of recognizing symptoms unique to particular disease processes, such as those specific to diabetes mellitus. One ancient Indian document specified the roles fulfilled by each member of a medical team, with the nurse responsible for knowledge of medication preparation in addition to "cleverness," devotion to the patient, and purity of both mind and body. Nurses are frequently referred to in Indian historical documents, although they were usually men or, in rare instances, older women. However, it is important to note that at this time in Indian history, nurses were already required to exhibit exceptional standards, skill at their craft, and a high level of integrity. Documentation from this period in India specified the characteristics required of a nurse (Donahue, 2010):

- Displaying appropriate behavior
- Clean
- Devoted to employer
- Kind
- Skilled at every type of service
- Clever in general
- Able to cook
- Skilled at bathing a patient
- Skilled at providing massage
- Able to assist a patient in walking and moving about
- Skilled at bedmaking
- Able to prepare or compound medications as needed
- Skilled at caring for a patient who had a difficult recovery

- Always willing to carry out any act, whether commanded by the physician or the patient

In this period in history, nursing as a vocation was predominantly comprised of males. However, after the third century A.D., the gradual entrance of women into nursing was affected primarily by three factors: the improvement in the social stature of women in the Roman Empire, the teachings of Christianity regarding the equality of people in service to God, and the requirement of Christians to continue the work of Christ with the neglected poor. As the Christian church began to assume care of the poor and the sick of the community, women as well as men began to share this task.

Among women, deaconesses and widows began to emerge as nurses and became the prototype for the modern community health nurse. Deaconesses worked equally with male deacons and were usually required to be unmarried or widowed. Their role as visiting nurses was carried out in addition to attending to the spiritual needs of their parishioners. Widows also served as visiting nurses for the poor and were usually required to swear a vow of chastity, leading to their ultimate development into nuns. A counterpoint to deaconesses and widows were the matrons of the Roman Empire who had converted to Christianity. Their positions of authority in society and considerable wealth allowed them to have the freedom to lay the foundation for community health nursing (Donahue, 2010). Paula of Actin, in particular, was an extremely wealthy and learned Christian widow believed to be the first to train nurses systematically and to teach nursing as an art rather than as merely a service to the poor. However, by that time a well-trained nurse was still considered to be one who not only cared for the sick but also cooked, cleaned, and waited on any other individuals in residence at the moment who might require service (Moses, 2011).

Transition to Secular Nursing

As the Middle Ages progressed, eventually the Reformation developed and a clear-cut religious division resulted, generating both a Catholic Church and Protestantism. In England more so than in any other country in Europe, monks and nuns were forced from monasteries, and hospitals and other facilities that had once been used to care for the poor and sick by religious orders were either closed or given over to other groups with less pure motives. For the first time, nursing began to be less associated with religion.

To fill the void produced by the lack of nuns and other women with similar religious dedications, women from the lowest levels of society were often recruited and assigned nursing duties to replace a certain amount of a prison sentence. Hospitals became severely utilitarian, and sanitary conditions were unknown. An 18th century hospital was described as having up to six patients stretched across the width of one bed. Patients never received bed baths, and it was standard practice for a patient with a highly contagious disease to be laid in the same bed with a patient who had a reasonably treatable illness, because the cause of infection was not understood at that point in history (Donahue, 2010).

It was at this time that men seemed to take their exit from nursing. After this period, nursing in Catholic countries was carried out by women in some type of religious order, whereas in Protestant countries nursing began to be seen as a female-dominated occupation. However, leadership of hospitals was almost always a male function, and virtually no authority was given to the women who provided oversight of the nurses hired to carry out the menial chores that were then considered to be "nursing." Because of the low character of many of the women who were acting as nurses at that time, an attempt was made to develop qualifications for women who sought to function as nurses in hospitals. The set developed by Thomas Fuller, an English physician, was as follows (Donahue, 2010):

- Middle-aged
- Healthy, particularly free from "vapors" and coughing
- Capable of being at the bedside throughout the course of the entire illness
- Ready to respond at the first call of the patient
- Capable of speaking very little, and then only in low tones, and able to walk softly
- Having keen eyes to observe any alteration in the patient's color, manner, or growth
- Able to do "everything the best way"
- Able to do everything quickly
- Clean in her habits
- Well-tempered and able to humor the sick person
- Cheerful and pleasant and never cross or sad
- Capable of observing the patient both night and day
- Not subject to practicing gluttony, drinking, or smoking
- Following the physician's orders carefully
- Childless (Table 1.1)

TABLE 1.1. Comparison of Qualifications for Nurses From the 1500s to the 1700s

QUALIFICATIONS FOR NURSES IN INDIA AFTER 1500	QUALIFICATIONS FOR NURSES DEVELOPED BY DR. THOMAS FULLER
Appropriate behavior	Middle-aged
Cleanliness	Healthy, particularly free from "vapors" and coughing
Devotion to employer	Capable of being at the bedside throughout the course of the entire illness
Kind	Ready to respond at the first call of the patient
Skilled at every type of service	Capable of speaking very little, in low tones, and walk softly
Clever in general	Having keen eyes to observe any alteration in the patient's color, manner, or growth
Able to cook	Able to do "everything the best way"
Skilled at bathing a patient	Able to do everything quickly
Skilled at providing massage	Clean in her habits

(continued on next page)

QUALIFICATIONS FOR NURSES IN INDIA AFTER 1500	QUALIFICATIONS FOR NURSES DEVELOPED BY DR. THOMAS FULLER
Able to assist a patient in walking and moving about	Well-tempered and able to humor the sick person
Skilled at bedmaking	Cheerful and pleasant and never cross or sad
Able to prepare or compound medications as needed	Capable of observing the patient both night and day
Skilled at caring for a patient with a difficult recovery	Not subject to practicing gluttony, drinking, or smoking
Always willing to carry out any act, whether directed by the physician or the patient	Following the physician's orders carefully
	Having no children

Emergence of Modern Nursing

Modern nursing had its genesis in the efforts of Theodor Fliedner, a Lutheran minister who revived the order of deaconesses after contact with the Moravians, who had revived the use of deaconesses in 1745. Recognizing the great need these individuals had filled in the health care community of the time, Pastor Fliedner founded a hospital and training center at Kaiserswerth, Germany, in 1836. By 1850, the renown of the Deaconess Institute had spread beyond the borders of Germany into other European countries, and Florence Nightingale chose to come there for instruction at that time (Wentz, 1936).

Miss Nightingale was born in 1820 into a wealthy English family who was progressive enough to see the benefits of a thorough education for both men and women. At a time when even wealthy women received only a rudimentary education, she was schooled in various languages as well as science and mathematics. As an adult traveling in Europe, she noted various facilities where nursing was taught in systematic curriculums, thus fueling her already burning desire to attain some type of life work that involves the care of others. Her parents objected to her affiliation with any hospital because of the terrible conditions that existed in these facilities at the time, with the worst such hospitals in England.

By 1854, the Crimean War had broken out, and English newspapers were filled with reports of the appalling care being provided to soldiers in English field hospitals. The care provided in French field hospitals was known to be far superior, primarily due to the efforts of the French Sisters of Charity, who had accompanied France's expedition to the Crimea in large numbers to care for the wounded. Miss Nightingale had previously become acquainted with England's secretary of war, who was so impressed with her and her desire to work with the sick and the dying that he wrote to her asking for her help in organizing the care of the English wounded in Turkey (Donahue, 2010).

By October 1854 Miss Nightingale had been appointed superintendent over the female nurses in the English field hospitals in Turkey and sailed for Scutari along with 38 nurses.

Upon arrival, she found 4 miles of beds holding approximately 3,500 wounded patients in a space designed for 1,700 men. The only light was given off by candles jammed into empty beer bottles, and an open sewer ran under the building. There was no water, soap, towels, knives or forks, or clothing for the patients and very little edible food. The death rate was slightly over 42%. To change the hospital from merely a storehouse for the dying into an area where the seriously ill and wounded could convalesce, Miss Nightingale opted to establish five kitchens for decent food preparation and a laundry as well as areas where recuperating soldiers could read and listen to music. In the evening, she frequently made rounds alone with her lantern to observe the progress of the most critical patients, acquiring the now famous title of "The Lady With the Lamp." Within six months of the implementation of the hygienic measures upon which Miss Nightingale insisted, the mortality rate in the hospital dropped to 2.2% (Donahue, 2010).

As a result of Florence Nightingale's growing fame from engineering the monumental change in English military health care and the gratitude she received from the British public, she achieved enough influence to develop a training program for nurses in a school devoted solely to this purpose. This was developed despite the objections of many English physicians who believed that such training was unnecessary because the nurse was essentially in the same position as a "housemaid" and therefore required no special training or instruction (Donahue, 2010).

Nursing During the Civil War

The development of nursing in America was a slow process, with the first nurses being servants, criminals, and paupers who cared for the sick. During the 17th and 18th centuries in America, nurses from various religious orders were asked to come in and reform hospitals that had become obstacles to a patient's recovery rather than assisting with the recovery process. However, this changed with Dorothea Dix. Miss Dix was the superintendent of female nurses for the Union Army during the Civil War and was given the authority to organize hospitals for the care of the wounded soldiers, appoint nurses to serve in such field hospitals, and oversee the distribution of supplies for the troops. Although not a trained nurse by profession, Miss Dix had a wealth of administrative and organizational skills acquired during her efforts 20 years earlier to create more humane living conditions for the mentally ill and criminals in America's prisons. Like Thomas Fuller a century earlier, Miss Dix developed a set of requirements for women seeking to obtain an appointment as a nurse (Donahue, 2010):

- Between ages 35 and 50
- Healthy and free of chronic diseases
- "Matronly," "good conduct," "superior" education, and "serious" personality
- Neat, orderly, and industrious
- Able to produce at least two references to attest to the candidate's character, morality, integrity, and ability to care for the sick
- Obedience and conformity with developed rules
- Able to serve in this capacity for at least three months, with preference given to those able to serve for longer periods (Tables 1.2 and 1.3)

TABLE 1.2. Comparison of Qualifications for Nurses From the 1700s to the 1800s

QUALIFICATIONS FOR NURSES DEVELOPED BY DR. THOMAS FULLER	QUALIFICATIONS FOR NURSES DEVELOPED BY DOROTHEA DIX
Middle-aged	Between ages 35 and 50
Healthy, free from "vapors" and coughing	Healthy and free of chronic diseases
Able to be at the bedside throughout the entire illness	Able to produce at least two references regarding character, morality, integrity, and ability to care for the sick
Cheerful and pleasant and never cross or sad	"Serious" personality
Able to do "everything the best way"	Able to serve for at least three months, preferably longer
Able to do everything quickly	Superior education
Able to speak very little, in low tones, and walk softly	Matronly
Having keen eyes to observe any alteration in the patient's color, manner, or growth	Neat, orderly
Clean in her habits	Good conduct
Well-tempered and able to humor the sick person	Industrious
Capable of observing the patient both night and day	Obedience and conformity with developed rules
Not subject to practicing gluttony, drinking, or smoking	
Ready to respond at the first call of the patient	
Following the physician's orders carefully	
Having no children	

TABLE 1.3. Comparison of Qualifications for Nurses From the 1500s to the 1800s

QUALIFICATIONS FOR NURSES IN INDIA AFTER 1500	QUALIFICATIONS FOR NURSES DEVELOPED BY DR. THOMAS FULLER	QUALIFICATIONS FOR NURSES DEVELOPED BY DOROTHEA DIX
Appropriate behavior	Middle-aged	Between ages 35 and 50
Cleanliness	Healthy, free from "vapors" and coughing	Healthy and free of chronic diseases
Devotion to employer	Able to be at the bedside throughout the entire illness	Able to produce at least two references regarding character, morality, integrity, and ability to care for the sick

QUALIFICATIONS FOR NURSES IN INDIA AFTER 1500	QUALIFICATIONS FOR NURSES DEVELOPED BY DR. THOMAS FULLER	QUALIFICATIONS FOR NURSES DEVELOPED BY DOROTHEA DIX
Kind	Cheerful and pleasant and never cross or sad	"Serious" personality
Skilled at every type of service	Able to do "everything the best way"	Able to serve for at least three months, preferably longer
Clever in general	Able to do everything quickly	Superior education
Able to cook	Able to speak very little, in low tones, and walk softly	Matronly
Skilled at bathing a patient	Having keen eyes to observe any alteration in the patient's color, manner, or growth	Neat, orderly
Skilled at providing massage	Clean in her habits	Good conduct
Able to assist a patient in walking and moving about	Well-tempered and able to humor the sick person	Industrious
Skilled at bedmaking	Capable of observing the patient both night and day	Obedience and conformity with developed rules
Able to prepare or compound medications as needed	Not subject to practicing gluttony, drinking, or smoking	
Skilled in caring for a patient with a difficult recovery	Ready to respond at the first call of the patient	
Always willing to carry out any act, whether directed by physician or patient	Following the physician's orders carefully	
	Having no children	

Another woman making a contribution to the war effort was **Clara Barton**, who independently organized and operated a huge war relief effort on behalf of the Union Army. She often used her own money to supply the recuperating soldiers with adequate food, clothing, bedding, and medical supplies. After the war, she learned of the existence of the International Red Cross and worked with this organization for several years. She soon began efforts to organize an American Red Cross, which did not come to fruition until 1882. Miss Barton served as the first president of the American Red Cross and gave her home to be its national headquarters (Barton, 1904).

The Confederacy also saw its share of women who made significant contributions to the developing profession of nursing, with **Sally Louisa Tompkins** and **Kate Cumming** being the most famous. Sally Louisa Tompkins was born into a wealthy Virginia family and responded to the Confederate government's call for the public to assist in caring for the wounded. Miss Tompkins founded Robertson Hospital in Richmond in 1861 and subsidized it primarily with her own funds. To prevent the hospital from being taken over by the military, Miss Tompkins convinced President Jefferson Davis to appoint her as captain of cavalry, making her the only woman to hold a commission in the Confederate Army. The military rank became invaluable to:

> Miss Tompkins because it came with a salary that could be used to defray the costs of operating the hospital along with the privilege of accessing medical supplies and government rations. By the time the hospital closed in 1865 at the conclusion of the war, Robertson Hospital had treated a total of 1,333 patients and sustained only 73 deaths, yielding a survival rate of 94.5%. This was remarkable at a time when the radical reforms of Florence Nightingale had occurred only a decade earlier. (Mathews County Historical Society, 2020)

In comparison with the southern born-and-bred Sally Louisa Tompkins, Kate Cumming was originally born in Scotland but moved with her family to Mobile, Alabama, in her youth and considered herself a southerner. After joining a party of 40 women who volunteered to journey to Corinth, Mississippi, to nurse the wounded, Miss Cumming became determined to seek a permanent position in a Confederate hospital. Despite the objections of her family and the public, by 1862 she had been appointed to the position of matron, or administrator, of the mobile field hospitals of Dr. Samuel Stout, the medical director for the Army of Tennessee. In her position of matron, Miss Cumming not only managed each mobile hospital's departments and supervised its workforce but also cooked, sewed, wrote letters, and foraged in the surrounding countryside for supplies. Her observations of the daily life of a confederate hospital during this time were chronicled in a diary that she kept and published after the war, one that gives us an invaluable picture of the hardships of that period and the strength of character of another of the great women of history who contributed to the nursing profession (Hilde, 2009).

Development of Schools of Nursing

The advent of the Civil War brought the woefully inadequate preparation of nurses in the United States to the forefront of the public's consciousness. Also, the public became more open to the idea of establishing formal training programs for nurses as more women from socially prominent families selected nursing as a vocation. The first formal instructional program for nurses is usually credited to Dr. Valentine Seaman, medical chief of New York Hospital. Dr. Seaman initiated a program of study for nurses in 1799 that continued until his death in 1817. This program became the framework for the entity that ultimately became Cornell University-New York Hospital School of Nursing (Engle, 1980).

As progress continued toward the development of formal training programs for nurses, the need for nurses to collaborate with female physicians in an effort to advance the professions of nursing and medicine became evident. Thus, in 1862 Drs. Marie Zakrzewska and Ednah Dow Cheney founded the New England Hospital for Women and Children. For more than 100 years, it was a teaching hospital for female physicians and later nurses run by an all-female staff that offered an education comparable with that received by male physicians. It was the first facility in the Boston area to offer obstetrics, gynecology, and pediatrics in one facility (Reiskind, 1995).

The first graduate of the facility's nurses' training program was Linda Richards in 1873. Considered to be the first trained nurse in America, Miss Richards, whose diploma is housed in the

Smithsonian Institution in Washington, DC, became the night supervisor at Bellevue Hospital and implemented major changes during her tenure: She insisted on the use of gas light at night rather than merely using a candle stub, she developed a system of charting and maintaining individual patient records, and she revealed the high mortality rate for new mothers who were dying of puerperal fever, a revelation that led to these patients being housed separately. After only a year Miss Richards became the superintendent of the Boston Training School, which was affiliated with Massachusetts General Hospital. Remarkably, she was able to combine administrative duties with actual bedside patient care during this time (Carnegie, 2000).

Another historically prominent figure who graduated from the nurses' training program at the New England Hospital for Women and Children was **Mary Eliza Mahoney**, the first African-American professional nurse. After working for the hospital since age 15, Miss Mahoney was admitted as a nursing student at age 33. At a time when the program admitted only one African-American student and one Jewish student into each class, she was one of only four students who completed the program out of an admitted class of 42 students. Working for many years as a private-duty nurse caring for patients in the New England area, Miss Mahoney went on to found the National Association of Colored Graduate Nurses. Today she is a member of the American Nurses Association's Nursing Hall of Fame and the National Women's Hall of Fame (Carnegie, 2000).

Nursing During World War I

Army and Navy Nurses Corp nurses who cared for casualties produced by World War I saw types of injuries that had never been produced before in wartime. The advent of both machine guns and poison gas generated horrific wounds that required new methods of treatment. The exact number of nurses who served in either Corps is uncertain because nurses tended to be grouped together into a general category of women who served in the war, but it is documented that by 1918 a total of 1,386 women were serving in the Navy Nurse Corps. The Red Cross estimates that almost 20,000 nurses were assigned to active duty during World War I and served either with the Army Nurse Corps, Navy Nurse Corps, U.S. Public Health Service, or the Red Cross overseas service. Most of these nurses served in the Army Nurse Corps (Budreau & Prior, 2008).

Many World War I nurses worked aboard trains that could evacuate up to 400 patients from front-line facilities in an effort to move them closer to embarkation points back to the United States. Each such train, also referred to as a *moving hospital*, was equipped with electric lights, steam heat, electric fans, and lavatories. However, these trains also complicated recovery, as the wounded had to contend with significant injuries as well as with the jolting motion, noise, and debris associated with long-distance train travel (Budreau & Prior, 2008).

One World War I–era nurse who became famous posthumously through her poignant letters was **Hedlen Fairchild**. Serving as one of 64 Pennsylvania nurses who joined the American Expeditionary Force after America entered the War in 1917, Miss Fairchild wrote of standing in mud above her ankles as she assisted in the operating suite. Her chief nurse described her and her fellow nurses as working 14-hour shifts with negligible amounts of rest. Tragically, Miss Fairchild would not live to see her wonderfully descriptive letters published. While working with the British Base Hospital in France, she volunteered for front-line duty at a casualty clearing station where she was exposed to mustard gas. She was found to have a large gastric ulcer and underwent surgery to repair it, but the surgery was not successful. Miss Fairchild died in January 1918 as a result of hepatic complications from the surgery that likely were worsened as a result of her exposure to the mustard gas (Patrick, 2011).

Nursing During World War II

As the prospect of war in Europe began to loom, the Army and Navy Nurse Corps had already been established and its members had served alongside the veterans of World War I. However, the federal government was slow to recognize the great need for nurses in the military until after the bombing of Pearl Harbor in December 1941. Earlier that year, in May, Congresswoman Edith Nourse Rogers had introduced the Women's Auxiliary Army Corps bill in an effort to mobilize the much-needed nurses as well as other female personnel to assist the war effort. Concurrently, by July 1942 Congress created the WAVES (Women Accepted for Volunteer Emergency Service) through the Women's Naval Reserve Act. This group of personnel was considered from their creation to be part of the Navy rather than an auxiliary. Ultimately, more than 140,000 women served in the Women's Army Corps and at least 100,000 served as Navy WAVES (Metropolitan State College of Denver, 2004). As a result of the valiant efforts of the nurses who served in World War II, fewer than 4% of the American soldiers who received treatment in the field or were evacuated died from either their wounds or disease. Reflecting the changing attitude in America toward the use of women in wartime as well as the great service being provided by the nurses in various theaters of war worldwide, by 1944 the Army was granting its nurses officers' commissions and full retirement privileges, along with pay equal to that of male counterparts and dependents' allowances. Between 1943 and 1948, the federal government provided free education to nursing students (Bellafaire, 2005).

On December 7, 1941, the day of the attack on Pearl Harbor, 82 Army nurses were stationed in Hawaii serving three Army medical facilities. Tripler Army Hospital was deluged with hundreds of casualties, and the wounded lay in the hallways awaiting their turn in the surgical suite. Medical supplies were in short supply as the wounded continued to pour into each facility, and sterile supplies ran out completely. Scissors were passed from one operating table to another, rags served double duty as both cleaning material and face masks for physicians and nurses, and operations were performed without the benefit of gloves. The chief nurse at Hickam Field, First Lieutenant Annie G. Fox, became the first Army nurse to receive the Purple Heart because of her example of calm, courage, and leadership during this ordeal (Bellafaire, 2005).

During most of 1941, Army nurses were increasingly sent to the Philippines as tension in that area increased. The Philippines were officially attacked by Japan on December 8, 1941, and consequently 45 nurses were sent from the island of Corregidor and Bataan to prepare two emergency hospitals. Of these hospitals, General Hospital 1 received more than 1,200 battle casualties requiring surgical procedures such as amputations within the first month. This hospital was bombed in March 1942 and received a direct hit, throwing patients from their beds. Body parts were found later that had been blown into the trees by the impact of the blast.

The dedication of the nurses serving in this area can be demonstrated by the heroism of those who stayed to care for the wounded. When it became clear that the island of Corregidor would fall, as many nurses as possible were evacuated to Australia. However, when the American forces surrendered to the Japanese on Corregidor, 55 Army nurses remained who had continued to care for the wounded at Malinta Hospital. These nurses were taken to an internment camp in Manila and remained prisoners of war until they were liberated by U.S. forces in 1945 (Doherty, 2000).

Along with starvation, tropical diseases, and deprivation of the very basic necessities of life, one group of 22 Australian nurses who had been shipwrecked in Indonesia faced being confronted and ultimately massacred by Japanese forces. The women were forced to march into the sea and then were shot as Japanese troops opened machine gun fire, despite the nurses having their Red Cross badges clearly evident. Of the 22 nurses, only one, Vivien Bullwinkel, received a wound that was not fatal and survived by pretending to be dead. She survived the massacre only to be captured and placed in an internment camp in Sumatra. However, in the internment camp Miss Bullwinkel was reunited with some of her nurse colleagues who had survived their shipwreck, and together they formed a support system that led to all except eight nurses surviving the camp internment (Doherty, 2000).

As World War II came to a close, many nurses who had been in military practice began to return to civilian lives, and a nursing shortage began developing rapidly. There was an increasing demand for nurses as soldiers returning to their prewar lives tried to cope with every type of injury, including loss of limbs and chronic wounds.

To remedy this situation, in 1952 the Cooperative Research Project in Junior and Community College Education for Nursing was initiated. This introduced the Associate Degree Nursing Program into the educational arena (Mahaffey, 2002).

Nursing During the Vietnam War

The Army Nurse Corps began its service in Vietnam in 1956 when three Army nurses arrived in Saigon to teach South Vietnamese nurses nursing procedures and nursing care techniques. This number of personnel expanded until December 1968, when 900 nurses were serving in 23 Army hospitals and a convalescent center that housed a combined total of more than 5,000 beds. The Army nurses in Vietnam were led by Colonel Mildred Clark and Colonel Anna May Hays, with Colonel Hays having been promoted to Brigadier General in 1970. Colonel Hays became the first nurse in American military history to attain general officer rank.

The nurses serving in Vietnam were on average ages 23 to 24 and were essentially new to nursing, with only 35% having had more than two years of experience as a nurse. They served a 12-month tour in Vietnam like all soldiers stationed there and typically worked six 12-hour days per week. Along with their assigned days on duty caring for military personnel, the Army nurses in Vietnam chose to continue to provide medical assistance to the Vietnamese civilians during their off hours. They conducted clinics where basic care could be administered, implemented sick calls at local orphanages, and led classes on child care for the residents of area villages (Norman, 1990).

The nurses stationed in Vietnam treated far more disease-related cases than battlefield injuries, specifically malaria, viral hepatitis, skin diseases, fevers, and diarrheal illnesses. Battlefield injuries were most often the result of assault rifles, rocket-propelled grenades, and booby traps. Multiple wounds tended to be seen when rapid-fire weapons were used. Blasts from mines resulted in severe injuries that were contaminated with debris and shrapnel, setting the stage for horrific infections. However, along with more traumatic injuries, the Vietnam era nurses also were witness to new advances in the treatment of casualties. Rapid evacuation by air, the availability of whole blood, well-established field hospitals, and advanced surgical techniques all combined to generate a mortality rate of 2.6% per thousand patients compared with the 4.5% experienced during World War II.

Vietnam-era nurses were renowned for their creativity and ability to improvise equipment in the harshest of conditions: Weights were made for traction by wrapping rocks in a Red Cross bag, a drinking straw was made from a piece of plastic gastrointestinal tubing, examination tables were built from discarded scrap lumber, and colostomy bags were formed from plastic dressing wrappers. Such ingenuity allowed the nurses to provide care for thousands of patients under the worst circumstances until the final Army nurse left the Republic of Vietnam in March 1973 (Norman, 1990).

Twenty-First Century Nursing

As nursing entered the 21st century, the profession was called to action for multiple crises, including the September 11, 2001, attacks, the War in Afghanistan, and the American Interventions in Iraq, Yemen, and Syria, to name only a few. However, the greatest challenge to nursing thus far in the 21st century has been the COVID19 pandemic. As nurses have risked their own safety to care for the multiple victims of the deadly virus, they conversely have had the advantage of seeing their roles expanded with the advent of telehealth. This tool, although used previously in health care, became widely used during the pandemic. It allowed nurses to address critical unmet health needs of patients and also set the stage for additional **doctor of nursing practice** (DNP)-prepared nurses to serve the public as primary care providers (Nikpour et al., n.d.).

Role Evolution in Modern Nursing

The RN student is one who is already seeking to assume a new role in the health care community, and as health care reform continues to make sweeping changes in modern medicine and the ways nursing care is delivered, the student may be in the position to not only assume a new role but to tailor that role to individual specifications. For example, the American Association of Colleges of Nursing (AACN; 2005) favors requiring nurses who choose to become **advanced practice nurses** such as nurse practitioners, nurse midwives, or certified registered nurse anesthetists to acquire a clinical doctorate, thus allowing them to be referred to as *DNPs*. According to the AACN, such a degree will allow practitioners who have acquired the degree to be on the same professional level as other disciplines, such as audiology, dentistry, medicine, pharmacy, physical therapy, and psychology, that have already required a practice doctorate for entry into practice as a health professional (Miller, 2008).

The doctor of nursing practice degree has proven to be one of both innovation and versatility and thus has lent itself to moving its graduates into teaching positions at the university setting. The degree is increasingly being recognized as much more than the clinical doctorate that it was once thought to be, and it is now discussed more for its advantages than its limitations. The National League for Nursing (2018) has called for collaboration between PhD-prepared nursing faculty and DNP-prepared faculty. This would help fill the shortage of nursing faculty, especially those with strong clinical backgrounds and leadership skills.

The clinical nurse leader (CNL) is another nursing role that may play a part in implementing health care reform. Initially, in 2003 the AACN proposed the CNL role as a way of responding to the increasing level of care required by the public and the changes in the health care environment. The CNL is intended to be capable of leading in all settings of health care delivery but is not intended to be an administrative or management position. The CNL is accountable for the health care outcomes for a specific set of clients through the use of nursing practice based on clinical research and is capable of functioning both as a provider and manager of care. The CNL may be called on to coordinate, delegate, or supervise care that is provided by the health care team (AACN, 2007).

The CNL role requires a thorough understanding of fiscal management, which allows the nurse to effectively manage resources, whether human, environmental, or material. He or she must be able to understand how to manage the budget for a nursing unit as well as how to develop a marketing plan and how to function in an organization (AACN, 2007). Measurement of the performance of the CNL will be determined by the extent to which this nurse can improve both clinical outcomes and cost outcomes for clients.

Nurses who are considering a career in academia or research may consider setting a goal for a PhD in nursing. This research-focused doctoral degree can set the foundation for a university teaching career but also can be useful in administrative roles or in a private practice setting. The PhD in nursing automatically conveys a certain amount of authority to the recipient because of the extensive preparation involved in obtaining the degree. The nurse who obtains this degree will be prepared to be influential regarding health care policy and nursing practice (https://nursing.careercast.com/article/5-career-benefits-phd-nursing).

Summary of Key Points in Chapter

This chapter described the historical development of nursing as a profession. Important concepts and individuals discussed are as follows:

- Edwin Smith Surgical Papyrus
- Provisions of the Mosaic Law and modern nursing
- Contribution of deaconesses and widows to development of modern nursing
- Florence Nightingale
- Dorothea Dix
- Clara Barton
- Sally Louisa Tompkins
- Kate Cumming
- New England Hospital for Women and Children
- Linda Richards
- Mary Eliza Mahoney

In addition, the efforts of nurses during wartime to care for patients were discussed, specifically in relation to World War I, World War II, and the Vietnam War. The evolution of the new roles of DNP and CNL and their relationship to the nursing community were discussed as well.

▶ Conclusion

Like many professions, the history of nursing has been a lengthy one, stretching from ancient times until the present day (Figure 1.1), where it continues to evolve. However, unlike other professions, it has played a part in literally every nation's development because of the universal need for well-being, the desire to be nurtured in a wholesome environment, and the importance of healing of body, mind, and spirit in an environment of safety and security. Nurses will continue to fulfill these needs for humankind worldwide as we move beyond the 21st century.

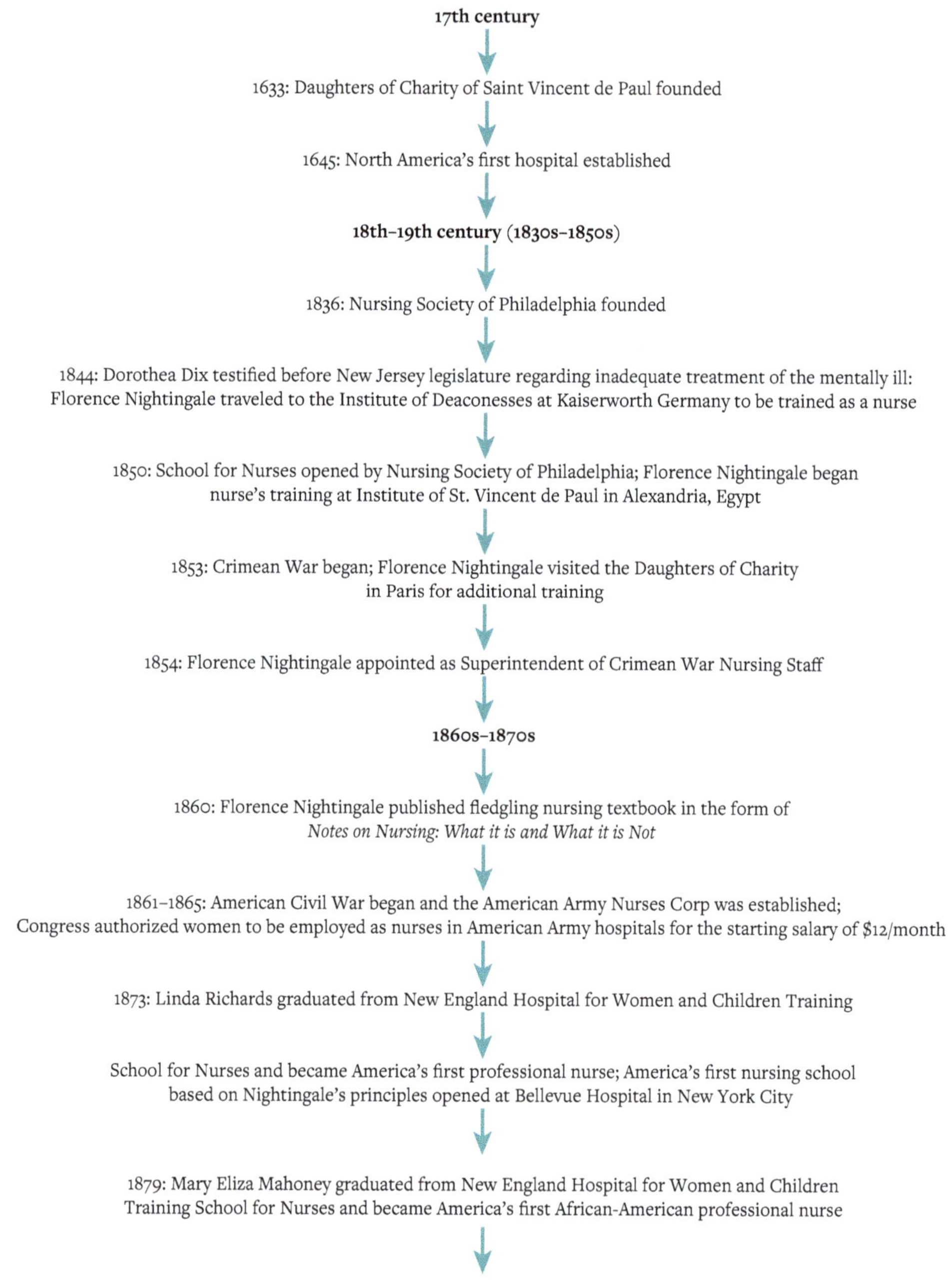

1880s–890s

1881: Clara Barton became first president of the American Red Cross

1886: First American nursing journal published

1893: Lillian Wald, founder of America's visiting nurses, began teaching home-based nursing classes in New York City; the Nightingale Pledge was first used by a graduating nursing class at Harper Hospital in Detroit Michigan

1897: American Nurses Association held its first meeting

1900s–1910s

1901: New Zealand became first country to regulate nurses nationally

1902: Ellen Dougherty of New Zealand became first registered nurse in the world; Lina Rogers Struthers hired as North America's first school nurse

1908: U.S. Navy Nurse Corps established

1909: University of Minnesota awarded first Bachelor's Degree in Nursing

1920s–1930s

1923: Yale School of Nursing became first autonomous American school of nursing; Mary Breckinridge founded Frontier Nursing Service

1938: Nurses Memorial in Arlington National Cemetery erected to honor World War I nurses

1940s and beyond

1942: U.S. Army nurses imprisoned in the Philippines

1949: U.S. Air Force Nurse Corps established

1956: Columbia University School of Nursing became first American university to grant a Master's Degree in a clinical nursing specialty

1965: First nurse practitioner role established at University of Colorado

1967: Dame Cicely Saunders established first hospice in London, England

1971: American hospice movement was established

1979: First nursing doctorate established at Case Western Reserve University

FIGURE 1.1. Timeline of Significant Events in Nursing History

Critical Thinking Questions

1. Review the dietary and hygienic teachings that are specific to the Mosaic Law. Which nursing practices used today can be traced back to these instructions?

    a. If the instructions of the Mosaic Law specific to dietary and hygienic practices were implemented today, do you believe the result would be successful? Give the rationale for your answer.

2. Review the characteristics of a nurse under Brahmanism in ancient India. Do you believe the modern-day nurse embodies any of these characteristics? If so, which ones?

    a. Do you believe the characteristics that were expected of nurses in the Brahmin-dominated society were realistic? Give the rationale for your answer.

3. Review the set of characteristics that were considered to be necessary for a nurse in India after 1500 as well as those specified for a nurse during the 17th century. Compare them and discuss how they are similar and different.

4. Compare and contrast the contributions of Dorothea Dix, Clara Barton, Sally Louisa Tompkins, and Kate Cummings to nursing during the American Civil War era.

5. Compare and contrast the contributions of Linda Richards and Mary Eliza Mahoney to the development of modern nursing. Do you believe some of the same obstacles these nursing pioneers faced still exist in nursing today? Be able to support your answer.

6. Compare and contrast the contributions of Helen Fairchild and Vivien Bullwinkel to the development of modern nursing. What coping methods do you believe these heroic nurses used to help them practice nursing under such terrible conditions?

Scenarios

1. Florence Nightingale used the outbreak of the Crimean War as an opportunity to take nursing much further along the route to becoming a respectable profession. What do you believe would be needed today to progress nursing further to becoming a profession that is entered equally by both men and women?

2. Compare and contrast the requirements for a nurse in India after 1500 with those specified by Thomas Fuller as well as those developed by Dorothea Dix. How did they change over that 300-year period of time, and how did they remain relatively unchanged?

3. Develop a set of qualifications to be a nurse in the 21st century. How do your requirements compare with those for an Indian nurse, those developed by Thomas Fuller, and those specified by Dorothea Dix?

4. Consider the hardships faced by nurses during the various wartime theaters of World War II. Do you believe today's modern nurse would be able to cope as well as these nurses did when faced with similar challenges? Be able to support your answer.

5. What preparation do you believe is needed for the modern nurse to be equipped to deal with a prisoner-of-war situation such as that faced by the nurses on the island of Corregidor during World War II?

6. How do you believe the role of the nurse changed from World War I to World War II? How do you believe the role of the nurse was affected by changes that occurred in modern medicine during this period of time?

7. Create a table that compares the hardships experienced, role(s) served, and circumstances under which nurses provided care in World War I, World War II, and the Vietnam War.

▸ NCLEX-Style Review Questions

1. Health-related instructions provided to the Israelites by the priestly tribe of the Levites included (select all that apply):
   a. selection of food that was in accordance with dietary requirements
   b. proper treatment of a woman during pregnancy and childbirth
   c. recognizing communicable disease so that the person could be put to death
   d. specific times for work, rest, and sleep during the course of each day

2. Characteristics required of nurses in India during the period in which Brahmanism was practiced included _______________:
   a. skill in caring for women
   b. skill in caring for children
   c. skill in bathing a patient
   d. skill in assisting with surgery

3. "Able to do everything the best way" is most likely considered a characteristic of a nurse during the time of:
   a. Thomas Fuller in the 18th century
   b. Brahminism-era India after 1500 B.C.
   c. Theodor Fliedner in the 19th century
   d. Florence Nightingale in the 19th century

4. "Clever in general" is most likely considered a characteristic of a nurse during the time of:
   a. Thomas Fuller in the 18th century
   b. Brahminism-era India after 1500 B.C.
   c. Theodor Fliedner in the 19th century
   d. Florence Nightingale in the 19th century

5. The individual who most effectively revived the Order of the Deaconesses was _______________:
   a. Dorothea Dix
   b. Florence Nightingale
   c. Theodor Fliedner
   d. Clara Barton

6. Florence Nightingale cared for wounded and dying soldiers during which war or military campaign?
   a. American Civil War
   b. Spanish-American War
   c. World War I
   d. Crimean War

7. The superintendent of female nurses for the Union Army during the Civil War was _______________:
   a. Dorothea Dix
   b. Florence Nightingale
   c. Kate Cumming
   d. Clara Barton

8. "Matronly with a serious personality" is a requirement for a female nurse from the set of qualifications developed by ______________:
   a. Dorothea Dix
   b. Florence Nightingale
   c. Kate Cumming
   d. Clara Barton

9. The American Red Cross was organized by ______________:
   a. Sally Louisa Tompkins
   b. Kate Cumming
   c. Clara Barton
   d. Dorothea Dix

10. The woman who founded a hospital and became appointed as captain of cavalry during the Civil War was:
    a. Sally Louisa Tompkins
    b. Kate Cumming
    c. Clara Barton
    d. Dorothea Dix

11. The first trained nurse in America is known to be:
    a. Ednah Dow Cheney
    b. Linda Richards
    c. Mary Eliza Mahoney
    d. Helen Fairchild

12. The nurse who became known as the first African-American trained nurse was:
    a. Ednah Dow Cheney
    b. Linda Richards
    c. Mary Eliza Mahoney
    d. Helen Fairchild

13. The nurses who coped with wounded transported on trains known as "moving hospitals" were most likely to have served during which wartime era:
    a. Civil War
    b. World War I
    c. World War II
    d. Vietnam War

14. Helen Fairchild is most closely associated with which era of wartime nursing?
    a. Civil War
    b. World War I
    c. World War II
    d. Vietnam War

15. A nurse who joined the Navy Nurse Corps when it was newly established was most likely to have served during which era of wartime nursing?
    a. Civil War
    b. Vietnam War
    c. World War II
    d. World War I

16. A nurse who was a member of the WAVES was most likely to have served during which era of wartime nursing?
    a. Civil War
    b. Vietnam War
    c. World War II
    d. World War I

17. The World War II–era nurse who was the first Army nurse to receive the Purple Heart was:
    a. Vivien Bullwinkel
    b. Annie G. Fox
    c. Mildred Clark
    d. Anna May Hays

18. The nurse who became the first nurse in American military history to attain general officer rank was:
    a. Vivien Bullwinkel
    b. Annie G. Fox
    c. Mildred Clark
    d. Anna May Hays

19. The doctor of nursing practice degree can most accurately be described as:
    a. an administrative or management position requiring knowledge of fiscal management
    b. preparation for the nurse to lead in all settings of health care delivery
    c. a clinical doctorate most likely used by an advanced practice nurse
    d. the ultimate degree for a nurse who wishes to provide instruction at the college level

20. The clinical nurse leader role can most accurately be described as:
    a. an administrative or management position requiring knowledge of fiscal management
    b. preparation for the nurse to lead in all settings of health care delivery
    c. a clinical doctorate most likely used by an advanced practice nurse
    d. the ultimate degree for a nurse who wishes to provide instruction at the college level

21. Arrange the following nursing leaders in order of their appearance in history:
    a. ____Helen Fairchild
    b. ____Mildred Clark
    c. ____Dorothea Dix
    d. ____Vivien Bullwinkel
    e. ____Linda Richards
    f. ____Sally Louisa Tompkins

22. As a registered nurse (RN), you are considering eventually moving into a career in academia. The best way for you to prepare yourself for this career move is to obtain a(n):
    a. DNP degree
    b. EdD in education
    c. PhD in nursing
    d. certification as a CNL

23. As a DNP-prepared RN, you are considering opening your own private practice. To expedite this occurring, you should plan to be comfortable utilizing:
    a. Medicaid billing
    b. leadership skills
    c. telehealth
    d. a team approach

Note Taker

I. Origins of nursing

A. Edwin Smith surgical papyrus

B. Brahmanism: characteristics of nurses

II. Transition to secular nursing

A. Thomas Fuller's qualifications of nurses

III. Emergence of modern nursing

A. Theodor Fliedner

B. Florence Nightingale

IV. Nursing during the Civil War

A. Dorothea Dix

B. Clara Barton

V. Development of Schools of Nursing

A. Linda Richards

B. Mary Eliza Mahoney

VI. Nursing during World War I

A. Helen Fairchild

VII. Nursing during World War II

A. Annie G. Fox

B. Vivien Bullwinkel

C. Associate degree nursing programs

VIII. Nursing during the Vietnam War

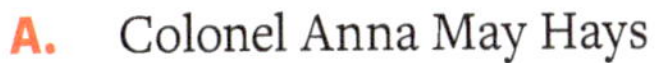

A. Colonel Anna May Hays

IX. Role of evolution in modern nursing

A. Doctor of nursing practice

B. Clinical nurse leader

References

American Association of Colleges of Nursing. (2022). *The state of doctor of nursing practice education in 2022*. https://www.aacnnursing.org/Portals/42/News/Surveys-Data/State-of-the-DNP-Summary-Report-June-2022.pdf

American Association of Colleges of Nursing. (2013). *Competencies and curricular expectations for clinical nurse leader education and practice*. https://www.aacnnursing.org/news-information/position-statements-white-papers/cnl

Barton, C. (1904). *A story of the Red Cross*. Appleton and Company.

Bellafaire, J. A. (2005). *The Army Nurse Corps in World War II*. http://www.history.army.mil/books/wwii/72-14/72-14.HTM

Budreau, L. M., & Prior, R. M. (2008). *Answering the Call, The U.S. Army Nurse Corps, 1917–1919, A Commemorative Tribute to Military Nursing in World War I*. Office of Medical History, Office of the Surgeon General, United States Army.

Carnegie, M. (2000). *Path we tread: Blacks in nursing* (3rd. ed.). Lippincott, Wilkins, and Williams.

Doherty, M. (2000). *Letters from Belsen 1945: An australian nurse's experiences with the survivors of war.* NSW College of Nursing.

Donahue, M. P. (2010). *Nursing: The finest art* (3nd ed.). Mosby.

Engle, R., Jr. (1980). Medical center archives. In New York Hospital Training School for Nurses (Cornell University-New York Hospital School of Nursing). http://www.med.cornell.edu/archives/history/timeline.html?name1=Historical+Timeline&type1=2Active

Five career benefits of a PhD in nursing. https://nursing.careercast.com/article/5-career-benefits-phd-nursing

Hilde, L. (2009). Kate Cumming. *Encyclopedia of Alabama.* http://www.encyclopediaofalabama.org/face/Article.jsp?id=h-1101

Mahaffey, E. (May 31, 2002). The relevance of associate degree nursing education: Past, present, future. *Online Journal of Issues in Nursing,* 7(2), Manuscript 2. www.nursingworld.org/ojin/MainMenuCategories/ANAMarketplace/ANAPeriodicals/OJIN/TableofContents/Volume72002/No2May2002/RelevanceofAssociateDegree.aspx

Mathews County Historical Society. (2020). Captain Sally Louisa Tompkins. https://www.mathewscounty-historicalsociety.org/

Metropolitan State College of Denver. (2004). Women in the military (military life). *The Women Army Corps.* Retrieved from http://www.mscd.edu/history/camphale/wim_001.html

Miller, J. (2008). The doctor of nursing practice: Recognizing a need or graying the line between doctor and nurse? *Medscape Journal of Medicine, 10*(11), 253.

Moses, A. (2011). St. Paula of Rome. *The Self-Ruled Antiochian Orthodox Christian Archdiocese of North America.* http://www.antiochian.org/node/17350

National League for Nursing. (2018). *Doctoral faculty collaboration in nursing education.* https://www.nln.org/docs/default-source/uploadedfiles/default-document-library/dnp-20183859c75c78366c709642ff00005f0421.pdf?sfvrsn=b96fab0d_0

Nikpour, J., Arrington, L., Michels, A., & Franklin, M. (n.d). *COVID-19 and the nursing profession: Where must we go from here?* https://healthpolicy.duke.edu/covid-19-and-nursing-profession-where-must-we-go-here.

Norman, E. (1990). *Women at war: The story of fifty military nurses who served in Vietnam.* University of Pennsylvania.

Nunn, J. F. (2008). A treatment that has stood the test of time for over three and a half millennia. JLL Bulletin. https://www.jameslindlibrary.org/articles/a-treatment-that-has-stood-the-test-of-time-for-over-three-and-a-half-millennia/

Patrick, B. K. (2011). *Army Nurse Helen Fairchild.* Military.com. http://www.military.com/Content/MoreContent?file=ML_fairchild_bkp

Reiskind, M. (1995). Hospital founded by women for women. *Jamaica Plain Historical Society.* https://www.jphs.org/

Wentz, A. (1936). *Fliedner the faithful.* Board of Publication of the United Lutheran Church in America.

CHAPTER 2

Nursing Theory

KEY TERMS

acculturation
conceptual framework
contextual stimuli
cultural awareness
cultural diversity
cultural universality
culturally congruent care
diagnostic operation
energy field
ethnicity
exploitation phase
extrapersonal stressor
focal stimuli
identification phase
interpersonal stressor
intrapersonal stressor
model
nursing theory
orientation phase
prescriptive operation
process
propositions
regulatory operation
residual stimuli
resolution phase
theory of goal attainment
theory of nursing systems
theory of self-care
theory of self-care deficit
theory of transcultural nursing
unitary human being

CHAPTER OBJECTIVES

Upon completion of the chapter, you will be able to:

1. Discuss the major assumptions of various nursing theories
2. Describe nursing models that are unique to specific nursing theories
3. Select a theory of nursing that can be applied in daily nursing practice
4. Compare and contrast the concepts of major nursing theories

Introduction to Nursing Theory

The nursing profession has a theoretical basis, meaning that the practice of professional nursing is based on a specific body of knowledge rooted in nursing theory. *Nursing theory* refers to a group of interrelated concepts and definitions that together describe a certain view of nursing. It is that rooting of nursing practice in a theoretical basis that creates the view of nursing as a profession. Nursing theory assists the nurse in the development of critical thinking, nursing judgment, and decision-making in patient care. Use of nursing theory can help the registered nurse (Chitty & Black, 2010):

- Organize patient data
- Analyze patient data
- Understand connections between patient data

- Determine priorities in patient data so the most important pieces of information are selected
- Use evidence to make appropriate clinical decisions
- Plan theoretically based nursing interventions
- Accurately predict the outcomes of nursing interventions
- Accurately evaluate the outcomes of nursing interventions

Nursing theories are primarily composed of processes, propositions, models, and conceptual frameworks. **Processes** are considered to be a series of actions, proposed changes, or functions that are implemented to bring about a specific result. **Propositions** are statements that explain relationships between the concepts used in a certain theory. In comparison, **models** are a documentation of the interaction that occurs between concepts and the patterns that result from that interaction. Finally, conceptual frameworks direct how these interactions occur. The **conceptual framework** defines the patient, the environment, health, and nursing, and this directs the way in which nursing care is delivered within the confines of the nursing process (Parker & Smith, 2010). Once the basic components of nursing theories are understood, the individual theories and the theorists who developed them can be studied.

Florence Nightingale's Theory of Nursing

Florence Nightingale is considered to be the first nursing theorist, proposing the following (McKenna, 2002):

- Nursing requires a spiritual "calling" to be practiced effectively.
- Nursing requires specific educational requirements and specific training to be implemented appropriately.
- Nursing is not synonymous with the practice of medicine.
- Nursing is both an art and a science.
- Nursing is most effectively practiced through altering the environment to produce optimal conditions for the patient.

Nightingale had high expectations for nurses even in the 19th century. She indicated in her writings that the nurse should closely observe the patient to note changes and accurately make judgments about the patient's condition. She proposed that nursing education should be a combination of both clinical and classroom instruction. Nightingale believed that because nursing required a spiritual calling, the nurse should be equipped to assist the patient who was experiencing spiritual distress through some level of health teaching and ultimately health promotion (Alligood & Tomey, 2009).

A significant part of Nightingale's theory was the belief that a patient's health was a direct result of their environment. She recognized how providing clean air and water, sanitation, light, and bathing could contribute to a patient's recovery from significant illness. She addressed the nurse's responsibility to not only feed the patient but also document the amount of food eaten and the patient's response to the diet served. Nightingale also proposed that excessive noise in hospitals should be addressed because of the importance of adequate rest to the recovering patient (Chitty & Black, 2010).

Specific assumptions are unique to Nightingale's theory of nursing but also form the basis for nursing theories that were developed in later years (see Table 2.1):

TABLE 2.1. Basic Concepts of Nightingale's Theory of Nursing

CONCEPT	DESCRIPTION
nursing	The nurse uses scientific principles and applies skill in observing patients' health and both reporting and documenting changes in health status. The nurse intervenes as necessary in order to facilitate recovery. Nursing requires a spiritual "calling." Nursing requires specific educational requirements and specific training. Nursing is not synonymous with medicine. Nursing is both an art and a science. Nursing involves altering the environment for optimal conditions.
person	Health equates with being "well" and with using every available resource to ensure a person lives life to the fullest. Both disease and illness can benefit the person by repairing damage that occurred when health problems were not addressed.
health	The nurse was believed to have primary control regarding the patient's recovery. The patient was seen as an individual.
environment	The environment is everything outside of the person that can affect both the ill person and the well individual. Nightingale wrote about the need for improved sanitary living conditions and hygiene, health problems caused by unsanitary conditions, and ways they could be remedied.

Source: Alligood, M., & Tomey, A. (2009). Nursing theory: Utilization and application *(4th ed.). Elsevier.*

Nursing: Nightingale believed the trained nurse used scientific principles in their work, applied skill in observing patients' health as well as reporting and documenting changes in the health status, and intervened as necessary to facilitate the recovery of the patient.

Person: Nightingale usually spoke of the individual as the patient. Although nurses were believed to have the primary control regarding patients' recovery because they were responsible for performing tasks for the patient and arranging the environment in such a way as to speed the recovery process, patients were seen as individuals. Nightingale instructed nurses to ask patients about their preferences regarding, for instance, mealtimes to give patients some small measure of control regarding their surroundings.

Health: Nightingale viewed health as being "well" and as using every available resource to make certain a person lived life to the greatest extent possible. She believed that both disease and illness could benefit the person by repairing damage that occurred when they did not address health problems. To maintain the health of the individual, she believed that control of the environment on the part of the nurse as well as social responsibility was necessary.

Environment: Nightingale viewed the environment as everything outside of the person that could affect the person both with an illness and without. She believed the poor of her day, who frequently lived in the most desperate of conditions, could benefit greatly from changes in their environments that would not only affect their bodies but also influence their minds. Nightingale essentially designed rural health care and wrote exhaustively on the need for improved sanitary living conditions and hygiene, the health problems that unsanitary conditions could cause, and ways to remedy such situations (Tomey & Alligood, 2010).

Hildegard Peplau's Theory of Nursing

Hildegard Peplau made great strides in promoting nursing professionalism through the use of credentialing as well as advanced practice nursing. However, her theory of nursing is remarkable on its own because of its contribution to the study of psychiatric nursing. Peplau identified the nurse-patient relationship as one consisting of four phases: orientation, identification, exploitation, and resolution (Tomey & Alligood, 2010). In the **orientation phase**, the client meets the nurse for the first time, with both being strangers. In this phase, the problem is defined and the type of service required by the patient is specified. The client will seek assistance, communicate any needs, ask questions, discuss any preconceptions, and share past experiences (Chinn & Kramer, 2010).

The **identification phase** of the nurse-patient relationship involves interdependent goal setting by the nurse and patient so that the **exploitation phase** can use professional resources to assist in designing problem-solving alternatives. This enables the individual to feel a part of the helping environment. As the relationship progresses into the **resolution phase**, the professional relationship with the nurse is terminated once the patient's needs have been met through collaboration between the nurse and the patient (Chinn & Kramer, 2010).

Peplau proposed that, during the course of the nurse-patient relationship, six different nursing roles can be assumed: stranger, resource person, teacher, leader, surrogate, and counselor. The nurse's time spent in these roles varies depending on the work setting (Tomey & Alligood, 2010). During the course of the nurse-patient relationship, the roles progress as follows (Chinn & Kramer, 2010):

Stranger: The nurse and the patient meet initially; the nurse is careful to generate an accepting trust-building environment.

Teacher: The nurse supplies knowledge for the patient in response to a need that has been identified or an interest the patient has communicated.

Resource person: The nurse supplies specific information for the patient in response to a new problem that has been revealed or a new situation that has occurred.

Counselor: This person helps the patient understand and incorporate the meaning of the patient's current life situation; provides guidance as needed and encourages the patient to make changes as needed.

Surrogate: The person in this role acts on the patient's behalf as an advocate.

Leader: The person holding this position helps the patient assume the maximum responsibility for meeting their treatment goals in a way that satisfies the collaboratively set goals of the patient and the nurse.

Peplau's theory of interpersonal relations focused on the nurse-patient relationship rather than spotlighting the patient alone, with nursing care seen as occurring within the boundaries of the nurse-patient relationship (Table 2.2). The therapeutic interpersonal relationship was viewed as having two goals (Chitty & Black, 2010):

1. Patient's survival
2. Patient's understanding of and learning from their health problems as new behavior patterns began to develop

TABLE 2.2. Peplau's Nurse's Roles in the Nurse-Patient Relationship

ROLE	DESCRIPTION	EXAMPLE
Stranger	The nurse and the patient meet initially; the nurse is careful to generate an accepting environment that is trust-building.	The nurse and patient meet for the first time, having previously been strangers.
Teacher	The nurse supplies knowledge for the patient in response to a need that has been identified or an interest that the patient has communicated.	The patient communicates that colon cancer runs in his family and he would like to learn how to incorporate additional fiber into his daily diet.
Resource person	The nurse supplies specific information for the patient in response to a new problem that has been revealed or a new situation that has occurred.	The patient communicates that she has been experiencing menstrual cycles that are heavier than usual.
Counselor	The counselor helps the patient understand and incorporate the meaning of the patient's current life situation; guidance is provided as needed; and the patient is encouraged to make changes as necessary.	The patient communicates that he has just been diagnosed with lung cancer.
Surrogate	The surrogate acts on the patient's behalf as an advocate.	At the patient's request, the nurse discusses a situation with the patient's family member that the patient cannot yet address.
Leader	The leader assists the patient in assuming the maximum responsibility for meeting treatment goals so that the collaboratively set goals of the patient and nurse are satisfied.	The nurse contracts with the patient for them to complete all of the sessions of outpatient therapy and lets it be the patient's responsibility to arrange their transportation to and from the clinic.

Sources: Alligood, M., & Tomey, A. (2009). Nursing theory: Utilization and application *(4th ed.). Elsevier; Reed, P., & Shearer, N.* (2011). Perspectives on nursing theory. *Lippincott, Williams, and Wilkins.*

Virginia Henderson's Theory of Nursing

Virginia Henderson is widely considered to be the 20th-century equivalent of Florence Nightingale. Her work as a nursing philosopher emerged at a time when there was a great need to determine the confines of nursing as a profession. She believed the definition of nursing could not be separated from the function of nursing, which she saw as assisting the person, whether they were ill or physically well, in performing the usual activities that contributed to their health or, if necessary, a peaceful death that they would perform without assistance if possible. Henderson believed the nurse was uniquely equipped to be a substitute for, helper to, or partner with the patient (Chitty & Black, 2010).

As part of her theory, Henderson emphasized the need to increase the patient's independence apart from the nurse so that after hospitalization, progress toward recovery would continue. In addition, the theory assumed that patients have an intrinsic desire to return to a state of health. Also, there was an assumption that nurses possessed both a willingness to serve the patient in the resumption of health and a willingness to devote themselves to the process around the clock, if the need presented itself (Parker & Smith, 2010).

Henderson believed 14 basic needs of the individual formed the basis for care delivered by the nurse. These needs formed a holistic view of the patient and also provided a multifaceted definition of the function of the nurse: to assist the patient who could not perform each of the 14 functions independently. Henderson described the 14 functions as

- Breathing
- Eating and drinking
- Elimination
- Mobility
- Sleeping/resting
- Dressing suitably for environmental temperature
- Maintaining body temperature
- Keeping body clean/grooming
- Avoiding endangering self or others in the environment
- Expressing thoughts and emotions
- Worshipping according to choice
- Receiving a sense of accomplishment from work
- Participating in recreational activities
- Learning about health and using available health facilities (Chitty & Black, 2010)

Virginia Henderson's theory of nursing included four primary concepts: the individual, the environment, health, and nursing. She saw the individual as

- Having basic needs that are all components of health
- Requiring assistance in the restoration of health
- Having an interrelationship between mind and body
- Being neither a client nor a consumer
- Being multifaceted, with physical, psychological, sociological, and spiritual needs

The environment of the individual was seen as the settings in which the person learns a pattern to be used for their day-to-day life as well as everything that affects the life of the person and their development. Henderson viewed health as the individual's ability to function without assistance and believed that nurses should actively engage in health promotion as well as disease prevention and the elimination of illness. Finally, she believed nursing provided a temporary assistance to the individual until they could return to independence (Parker & Smith, 2010). Table 2.3 shows the basic concepts of Henderson's theory of nursing.

TABLE 2.3. Basic Concepts of Henderson's Theory of Nursing

CONCEPT	DESCRIPTION
individual	The individual: • has basic needs that are all components of health • requires assistance in the restoration of health • has an interrelationship between mind and body • is neither a client nor a consumer • is multifaceted, with physical, psychological, sociological, and spiritual needs
environment	The environment consists of: • the settings in which a person learns a pattern for their day-to-day life • everything that affects the life of the person and their development
health	Health is the individual's ability to function without assistance.
nursing	Nursing provides a temporary assistance to the individual until they can return to independence. The nurse should actively engage in health promotion, disease prevention, and elimination of illness.

Source: Parker, M., & Smith, M. (2010). Nursing theories and nursing practice. *(3rd ed.) F. A. Davis.*

Ida Orlando's Theory of Nursing

Ida Orlando was one of the first nursing theorists to write extensively about the nursing process and the nurse-patient relationship. She believed the role of the nurse was to assess and ultimately meet the patient's immediate need for assistance. She believed the patient's presenting behavior was indirectly a call for assistance, although the help needed from the nurse might actually be different from that originally anticipated. For this reason, it is the nurse's responsibility to explore with patients the meaning of their behavior. This can best be done by using the nurse's perception about the patient's behavior, thoughts about the perception, or feelings derived from those thoughts.

There are four primary dimensions to Orlando's theory of nursing (Chinn & Kramer, 2010):

1. Distress: Experienced by the patient who has unmet needs.
2. Nursing role: To assess the patient's unmet needs and meet their immediate need for assistance. The nurse should recognize the patient's behavior may not, in fact, represent the true need that is occurring; thus, the nurse should validate their understanding of the unmet need with the patient.
3. Nursing actions: Designed to directly or indirectly provide for the patient's immediate needs.
4. Outcome: Change in the behavior of the patient indicating either a relief from immediate distress or an unmet need; can be noted both through verbal and nonverbal communication with the patient.

Apart from these four dimensions, other concepts unique to Orlando's theory include the following (Chinn & Kramer, 2010):

- Nursing: Viewed as being responsive to the individual who is experiencing a sense of helplessness or is anticipating that such helplessness will occur
- Health: Seen as a sense of well-being and comfort, with needs being fulfilled
- Human being: Considered to be a developmental being with needs
- Nursing client: Person under medical care who either cannot fulfill their medical needs or cannot carry out medical treatment without assistance from the nurse
- Nursing problem: Distress experienced by the nursing client; the distress may be caused by physical limitation, adverse reactions to the nursing client's environment, or experiences that can prevent the person from being able to make others aware of their needs
- Nursing process: An interaction of the patient's behavior, the nurse's reaction to that behavior, and nursing actions that are chosen for the benefit of the nursing client

Orlando's theory focused to the greatest degree on understanding problematic situations in which the nurse recognizes the patient is demonstrating behavior that is a cue for assistance. The patient's behavior will in turn generate a response from the nurse, a unique reaction that consists of the nurse's perceptions, feelings evoked, and the nurse's past experiences and acquired knowledge. The nurse and patient will need to communicate to determine the meaning of the patient's behavior and the help required. Once the patient's situation has been made clear, it will no longer be considered problematic; once the patient's most pressing needs have been identified and resolved, the patient's situation will improve, and a new equilibrium will develop (Alligood & Tomey, 2009).

Regarding the significance of Orlando's theory, Chitty & Black (2010) noted that it is very useful as a theory to be implemented in practice. It specifies how nursing clients can be involved in the decision-making process of the nurse and can guide interactions to yield predictable outcomes. Nurses can use the theory as they individualize care for each patient. This can be done by paying attention to the nursing client's behavior, carefully verifying ideas that the nurse derives from interaction with the client, and identifying client needs that appear to be of most concern to the individual (Chitty & Black, 2010). Table 2.4 summarizes the basic concepts of Orlando's theory.

TABLE 2.4. Basic Concepts of Orlando's Theory of Nursing

CONCEPT	DESCRIPTION
distress	Experienced by the patient who has unmet needs
nursing role	To assess the patient's unmet needs and meet their immediate need for assistance; the nurse should recognize that the patient's behavior may not represent the true need that is occurring, and therefore the nurse's understanding of the patient's unmet needs will require validation
nursing actions	Designed to provide for the patient's immediate needs
outcome	Change in the behavior of the patient indicating either relief from immediate distress or an unmet need
nursing	Viewed as being responsive to the individual who is experiencing a sense of helplessness

CONCEPT	DESCRIPTION
health	Seen as being a sense of well-being and comfort with needs being fulfilled
human being	Considered to be a developmental being with needs
nursing client	Person under medical care who either cannot fulfill medical needs or cannot carry out medical treatment without assistance from the nurse
nursing problem	Distress experienced by the nursing client; may be caused by physical limitation, adverse reactions to the nursing client's environment, or experiences that can prevent the person from being able to make others aware of the nursing client's needs
nursing process	An interaction of the patient's behavior, the nurse's reaction to that behavior, and nursing actions that are chosen for the benefit of the nursing client

Source: Chinn, P., & Kramer, M. (2010). Integrated theory and knowledge development in nursing. *Elsevier.*

Martha Rogers' Theory of Nursing

Rogers' theory of unitary human beings can be a difficult one for the registered nurse to grasp because of its complexity. Rogers was greatly influenced by the theory of relativity of Einstein, and her work also can be compared with von Bertalanffy's general system theory (Tomey & Alligood, 2010). Rogers' theory is particularly important because of its emphasis on nursing as both an art and a science (Table 2.5).

TABLE 2.5. Basic Concepts of Rogers' Theory of Nursing

CONCEPT	DESCRIPTION
unitary human being	• an integration of the human being and environment • human beings are one with the universe • the unitary human being cannot be separated from the environment
nursing	• purpose is to identify and examine the unitary human being • nursing should support the patient as the person progresses through life and ultimately achieves maximum potential for health
energy field	• basic unit of both the living and nonliving entities in the universe • energy fields vary constantly in intensity, density, and extent • there were no boundaries that prevent energy from flowing between energy fields • human energy and the environmental field are involved in a constant exchange of energy
health	• defined by the patient • the nurse should assist the patient in moving toward the patient's definition of health

(continued on next page)

CONCEPT	DESCRIPTION
scope of nursing	includes: • maintenance of health • promotion of health • prevention of disease • formulation of nursing diagnosis • development of nursing intervention • actions for rehabilitation

Source: Alligood, M., & Tomey, A. (2009). Nursing theory: Utilization and application (4th ed.). *Elsevier; Reed, P., & Shearer, N.* (2011). Perspectives on nursing theory. *Lippincott, Williams, and Wilkins.*

Rogers viewed nursing as being synonymous with a body of knowledge and a learned profession that must be based on scientific evidence. Such scientific knowledge should be used to improve the day-to-day existence of the **unitary human being**, which Rogers defined as being an integration of the human being and their environment (Tomey & Alligood, 2010).

Rogers' definition of the unitary human being is a complex one, in that she described the human being and the environment as energy fields greater than the sum of their parts. The concept is that nursing has as its purpose to both identify and examine the unitary human being. Rogers believed that nursing should support the patient as they progress through life and subsequently achieves maximum potential for health. The patient defines for themselves what health means, and therefore the nurse should assist the patient in moving toward that goal. She saw the scope of nursing as consisting of (Tomey & Alligood, 2010):

- Maintenance of health
- Promotion of health
- Prevention of disease
- Formulation of nursing diagnosis
- Development of nursing intervention
- Actions for rehabilitation

Some of Rogers' most complex ideas centered around the "unitary human being." She believed human beings are one with the universe, and subsequently the unitary human being cannot be separated from their environment. She further proposed a basic unit of both living and nonliving entities in the universe, which she referred to as the ***energy field***, and these energy fields were constantly varying in intensity, density, and extent. She believed there were no boundaries to prevent energy from flowing between energy fields, and the human energy and the environmental field were involved in a constant exchange of energy (Reed & Shearer, 2011).

Despite its complexity, Rogers' theory has relevance for the modern healthcare delivery system because of its emphasis on the inability to separate the patient's experience from their very existence as a human being. This is important in 21st-century health care, where the emphasis is more on the overall continuum of care and much less on periodic episodes of illness and treatment. Her theory's emphasis on nursing, which is based on scientific knowledge that can subsequently guide nursing practice, can be argued as the forerunner of the modern emphasis on evidence-based nursing practice (Tomey & Alligood, 2010).

Sister Callista Roy's Theory of Nursing

Sister Callista Roy's theory of nursing is based on adaptation and human adaptive behavior. Roy is currently a member of the order of Sisters of Saint Joseph of Carondelet, and her theory shows that influence in her focus on the human being as a biopsychosocial system that is constantly trying to cope with the demands placed by environmental stimuli. Roy proposed that when the individual can adapt effectively to the demands of environmental stimuli, the person can maintain integrity, conserve their energy, and ultimately promote their own survival, growth, and reproduction as a human system. Recognizing this, the registered nurse will assess the patient's adaptive behavior, develop nursing diagnoses to guide development of goals and nursing interventions to promote adaptation, and ultimately modify the environment to facilitate adaptation of the patient (Chitty & Black, 2010).

Roy believed the patient is constantly interacting with an environment that is also constantly changing. To cope with the constant change in the environment, the person must use both inborn mechanisms of coping and acquired mechanisms; these may be biological, psychological, or social in nature. The person's adaptation to environmental change is directly related to the stimulus to which they are exposed and their adaptation level. The adaptation level consists of a zone that indicates a range of stimuli that will produce a positive response in the individual. In turn, four modes of adaptation can be used by the individual: physiological needs, self-concept, role function, and interdependence (Reed & Shearer, 2011; Table 2.6).

TABLE 2.6. Basic Concepts of Roy's Theory of Nursing

CONCEPT	DESCRIPTION
stages of the nursing process	1. assess behaviors produced from the four adaptive modes 2. assess the stimuli for the behaviors that are produced and determine if they are: • focal, or those that immediately confront the patient • contextual, or all other stimuli present that will contribute to the effect of the focal stimuli • residual, or environmental factors that have effects that have not been determined in a specific situational adaptation 3. determine a nursing diagnosis reflective of the person's current adaptive state 4. set goals to promote the process of adaptation 5. implement interventions that will manage the stimuli and subsequently promote adaptation 6. evaluate if adaptive goals have been met through manipulation of stimuli rather than through manipulation of the patient
adaptation	considered to be the goal of nursing
person	• functions as an adaptive system • biopsychosocial being who is constantly interacting with the changing environment
environment	synonymous with stimuli, focal, contextual, or residual
health	considered to be the outcome of adaptation
nursing	promotes both health and adaptation

Source: Reed, P., & Shearer, N. (2011). Perspectives on nursing theory. *Lippincott, Williams, and Wilkins.*

Roy's theory departs from other theoretical proposals of nursing in her stages of the nursing process. She proposed the following six stages (Tomey & Alligood, 2010):

1. Assess behaviors produced from the four adaptive modes.
2. Assess the stimuli for the behaviors that are produced and determine if they are focal, contextual, or residual. **Focal stimuli** immediately confront the patient, **contextual stimuli** are all other stimuli present that contribute to the effect of the focal stimuli, and **residual stimuli** are environmental factors that have effects not determined in a specific situation.
3. Determine a nursing diagnosis reflective of the person's current adaptive state.
4. Set goals to promote the process of adaptation.
5. Implement interventions that manage the stimuli and subsequently promote adaptation.
6. Evaluate if adaptive goals have been met through manipulation of stimuli rather than through manipulation of the patient.

Specific concepts are considered to be unique to Roy's theory (Reed & Shearer, 2011):

- Adaptation: Considered to be the goal of nursing
- Person: Functions as an adaptive system; biopsychosocial being who is constantly interacting with the changing environment
- Environment: Synonymous with stimuli, focal, contextual, or residual
- Health: Considered to be the outcome of adaptation
- Nursing: Promotes both health and adaptation

Imogene King's Theory of Nursing

Imogene King is significant to nursing theory because of her **theory of goal attainment**. She proposed that nursing is a process through which the nurse and the client interact to develop a perception of each other and the client's situation and, as a result, develop goals for the client and collaborate on a means to achieve those goals. King consistently referred to the patient in her theory as "the client" (McElwen & Wills, 2018).

King's theory proposed that the nurse's focus was on issues of importance to the client; this focus was such a priority it was likely to prevent mutual goal setting from occurring. King believed each individual had multiple interpersonal relationships as well as three interacting systems, which she labeled *personal*, *interpersonal*, and *social*. These interacting systems together formed a framework that allowed the individual client to be seen in their entirety (Chitty & Black, 2010):

- The personal system provided an understanding of the client, both personally and within themselves.
- The interpersonal system provided an understanding of the interaction and transactions that can occur between multiple persons.
- The social system provided an understanding of social contacts with individuals in settings such as the workplace or school.

Whereas the previously mentioned theory of Virginia Henderson focused on the needs of the patient, King's theory focused on goal attainment both for and by the client. King believed nursing care for the client was guided by the personal, interpersonal, and social systems. The client's personal system caused the registered nurse to observe the client's perceptions, the interpersonal system caused the nurse to observe the client's multiple roles in their life as well as the stressors they experienced while interacting in each role, and the social system caused the nurse to note influences on the client's decision-making capabilities. King found interaction with the client to be of particular importance in the goal attainment theory and believed that specific steps in the communication process occurred as the client moved from a first encounter with the nurse until the desired goal was achieved. Identified as progressing in difficulty, the steps were labeled as follows:

- Perception
- Judgment
- Action
- Reaction
- Interaction
- Transaction

King also believed that progressive difficulty of the steps required an increasing level of involvement between the nurse and the client so that the nurse could achieve a comprehensive understanding of the goals of the client to appropriately plan and provide nursing care. This underscored the importance of goals being set on a collaborative basis between nurse and client (Chitty & Black, 2010).

King's theory of goal attainment viewed the nursing process as consisting of four stages: assessment, planning, implementation, and evaluation. In the assessment stage, the perceptions of the nurse and client are developed, mutual communication occurs, and interaction develops. In the planning stage, decisions are made about goals, and there is mutual agreement regarding the means used to attain those goals. During the implementation stage, transactions are made, and the subsequent evaluation stage determined if the goal was attained; if attainment did not occur, an investigation ensued to discover the reason (Alligood & Tomey, 2009).

Several primary concepts are considered to be intrinsic to King's theory:

- Nursing's goal is to help the client maintain their health so the individual can function in their role; nursing is an interpersonal process that is influenced by both the nurse and the client's perceptions. Nursing is a process that consists of action, reaction, interaction, and transaction.
- The individual is made up of an open system that is in transaction with the environment, meaning the client cannot be separated from their environment; the individual has a spiritual component and can think, use language, make choices, and choose from several courses of action; each individual is different in their wants, needs, and goals; is unique, holistic, and of worth; is able to think rationally; and can participate in decision-making in most instances.

- Health is considered to be a dynamic state in the individual's life cycle; thus, illness is considered to be an incident that interferes with the smooth progression of that life cycle.
- Environment for the client is constantly changing, and the individual constantly interacts with their environment to maintain a state of health; it is the interaction with the environment that influences each individual's adjustments to their life and state of health (Tomey & Alligood, 2010).

Table 2.7 summarizes the basic concepts of King's theory.

TABLE 2.7. Basic Concepts of King's Theory of Nursing

CONCEPT	DESCRIPTION
nursing	• has as its goal to help the client maintain health so that the individual can function in their role • is an interpersonal process that is influenced by perceptions of both the nurse and the client • is a process that consists of action, reaction, interaction, and transaction
individual	• is made up of an open system that is in transaction with the environment • the client cannot be separated from the environment • the individual has a spiritual component, can think, use language, make choices, and choose from multiple courses of action • each individual is different in their wants, needs, and goals; is unique, holistic, and of worth; is able to think rationally; and is able to participate in decision-making
health	• health is a dynamic state in the individual's life cycle • illness is an incident that interferes with the smooth progression of that life cycle
environment	• environment for the client is constantly changing • the individual constantly interacts with the environment to maintain a state of health • the interaction with the environment influences each individual's adjustments to the person's life and state of health

Source: Alligood, M., & Tomey, A. (2009). Nursing theory: Utilization and application (4th ed.). *Elsevier.*

Dorothea Orem's Theory of Nursing

Dorothea Orem was a nursing theorist who was a proponent of individuals being self-reliant and responsible for the health care of themselves and their family members. Orem actually designed three theories that involved self-care, self-care deficit, and the nursing system that fit together to form a larger theory known as the self-care deficit theory (Alligood & Tomey, 2009). The theory of self-care described why individuals choose to care for themselves and how they implement the care. The theory of self-care deficit explained why individuals can be helped through nursing and also described how such care can be beneficial. The theory of nursing systems proposed relationships that must be both developed and maintained in order for nursing to be implemented and attempted to explain the nature of these relationships (Tomey & Alligood, 2010).

Orem's theory of nursing focused on the capacity of the patient to provide self-care and the process of developing nursing interventions to fulfill the individual's unmet needs for self-care. The theory proposed that the patient has a self-care deficit consisting of the degree to which they are unable to provide self-care. Because of this self-care deficit, the nurse will need to regulate the nursing system, which consists of various relationships. Therefore, an overriding assumption of the theory is that the ordinary individual in modern society has a need to be in control of their own life (Chitty & Black, 2010).

Orem further proposed that the nurse should develop appropriate care for the individual through three types of operations: diagnostic, prescriptive, or regulatory. A **diagnostic operation** establishes the nurse-patient relationship and determines the individual's ability to provide self-care. The patient's ability to provide effective self-care will be assessed by the nurse to determine a baseline and measure the extent to which the patient has a limitation in providing their own self-care. These limitations are documented as self-care deficits. In comparison, **prescriptive operations** are used in a planning stage when the nurse confirms with the patient that the baseline assessment is accurate and that a plan of care is developed. Finally, in **regulatory operations**, the nurse designs and generates a system for nursing care for the patient that can range from completely compensatory, providing the highest level of care for the patient with little if any ability to provide self-care, to supportive or educational, providing assistance to the individual who has the ability to provide self-care but needs additional knowledge (Chitty & Black, 2010).

Some major assumptions are unique to Orem's theory of nursing (Table 2.8):

- Nursing is considered to be an art, a helping service, and a technology; the goal of nursing is to assist the individual in becoming capable of meeting their own self-care needs.
- Health is considered to be both structural and functional soundness; includes every quality that makes a person human.
- Human being is considered to have universal and developmental needs and to be capable of self-care on a continuous basis.
- A nursing problem occurs when there is a deficit in a universal, developmental, or health-derived or health-related condition (Chinn & Kramer, 2010).

TABLE 2.8. Basic Concepts of Orem's Theory of Nursing

CONCEPT	DESCRIPTION
nursing	• considered to be an art as well as a helping service and a technology • goal is to assist the individual in becoming capable of meeting the person's own self-care needs
health	• considered to be both structural and functional soundness • includes every quality that makes a person human
human being	• considered to be a being with universal as well as developmental needs • capable of self-care on a continuous basis
nursing problem	• occurs when there is a deficit in a universal, developmental, or health-derived or health-related condition

Source: Chinn, P., & Kramer, M. (2010). Integrated theory and knowledge development in nursing. *Elsevier.*

Betty Neuman's Theory of Nursing

Betty Neuman's theory of nursing is a system theory that has its roots in stress theory and the mental health community. Neuman proposed that each person is a system, meaning a group of characteristics and factors contained within a specific range of responses that may occur, and these factors and responses are in turn housed within a basic structure. Each person (usually referred to as a *client* in Neuman's theory) has developed a range of responses to the environment that is considered to be normal for their system. A deviation from the client's usual state of health is noted by determining the responses to the environment are no longer capable of protecting them from stressors. Within each client is a set of internal resistance factors that seek to stabilize them as a system and return that person to their usual state of wellness. The client as a system is in a state of homeostasis when there is a constant and ever-changing process of input, output, feedback, and subsequent compensation in response (McElwen & Wills, 2018).

Neuman's theory of nursing has specific concepts that are unique to it (Table 2.9):

TABLE 2.9. Basic Concepts of Neuman's Theory of Nursing

CONCEPT	DESCRIPTION	EXAMPLE
human being	consists of a client system with multiple layers; each layer is composed of five subsystems: 1. physiological 2. psychological 3. sociocultural 4. spiritual 5. developmental	
environment	the total internal and external forces that interact with a client	the internal environment is within the client; external environment is outside the client
health	synonymous with wellness	
nursing	concerned with all of the variables that affect the client's response to a stressor	
intrapersonal stressors	internal stressors that occur within the boundaries of the client's system	various disease processes
interpersonal stressors	those that occur in the external environment outside of the client system but close to the system boundaries	this could include client's multiple roles in his family and relationships with friends
extrapersonal stressors	those that occur in the external environment outside of the client system but farther away from the system boundaries	this could include client's employment status as well as various resources available to the client in the community

Source: Alligood & Tomey, 2009; McElwen & Wills, 2018

- Human being: Consists of a client system with multiple layers. Each layer is composed of five subsystems:
  1. Physiological
  2. Psychological
  3. Sociocultural
  4. Spiritual
  5. Developmental
- Environment: The total internal and external forces that interact with a client. The internal environment is within the client, whereas the external environment is outside the client.
- Health: Seen as being synonymous with wellness.
- Nursing: Viewed as being concerned with all variables that affect the client's response to a stressor (McElwen & Wills, 2018).

Neuman's theory of nursing focuses in large part on stressors that can influence the stability of the client system. Such stressors can be classified as intrapersonal, interpersonal, or extrapersonal. **Intrapersonal stressors** are the internal stressors that occur within the boundaries of the client's system, such as various disease processes. **Interpersonal stressors** are those that occur in the external environment outside of the client system but close to the system boundaries. This could include the client's multiple roles in their family and relationships with friends. Finally, **extrapersonal stressors** occur in the external environment outside of the client system but farther away from the system boundaries. This could include the client's employment status as well as various resources available to the client in the community (Alligood & Tomey, 2009).

Jean Watson's Theory of Human Science and Human Caring

Watson's theory of human science and human caring focuses on the practice of caring and assumes that it is central to nursing. Caring is viewed as being complementary to the science of caring. A caring environment is considered to be one that offers the individual the development of potential while allowing them to choose the best action for themselves at a specific time. Caring accepts the individual as they are now as well as what they may become. Effective caring is seen as promoting health and also the growth of the individual or the family. Watson proposes that the core of the theory of caring is that humans cannot be separated from self, other, nature, and the workforce. Caring consists of "carative factors" that will result in the satisfaction of specific human needs. The carative factors are considered to be as follows:

1. Embrace: incorporating altruistic values and practicing loving kindness with the self and others.
2. Inspire: embracing faith and hope and honoring others
3. Trust: nurturing individual beliefs, personal growth, and practices
4. Nurture: developing helping, trusting, and caring relationships
5. Forgive: accepting positive and negative feelings by authentically listening to another person's story
6. Deepen: utilizing scientific problem solving methods for caring decision-making

7. Balance: teaching and learning to address individual needs, readiness, and learning styles
8. Co-create: developing a healing environment for the physical and spiritual self that respects human dignity
9. Minister: addressing basic physical, emotional, and spiritual human needs
10. Open: to mystery and allowing miracles to enter (Psych-Mental Health Hub, n.d.)

TABLE 2.10. Basic Concepts of Watson's Theory of Nursing

CARATIVE FACTOR	DESCRIPTION
embrace	incorporating altruistic values and practicing loving kindness with the self and others
inspire	embracing faith and hope and honoring others
trust	nurturing individual beliefs, personal growth, and practices
nurture	developing helping, trusting, and caring relationships
forgive	accepting positive and negative feelings by authentically listening to another person's story
deepen	utilizing scientific problem-solving methods for caring decision-making
balance	teaching and learning to address individual needs, readiness, and learning styles
co-create	developing a healing environment for the physical and spiritual self that respects human dignity
minister	addressing basic physical, emotional, and spiritual human needs
open	to mystery and allowing miracles to enter

Source: Psych-Mental Health Hub. (n.d.). Jean Watson theory of human science and human caring. https://pmhealthnp.com/jean-watson-theory-of-human-science-and-human-caring/Madeleine Leininger's Theory of Nursing

Madeleine Leininger's primary contribution to theoretical nursing was the theory of nursing known as ***transcultural nursing***. She based her ideas on principles unique to the science of anthropology. After recognizing the world was rapidly becoming one in which humans would have to function multiculturally, she proposed that nursing was failing to provide nurses with adequate cultural knowledge. Leininger believed that culture is learned, is passed from one generation to the next, and can be observed in a person's actions, words, behavioral rules, and symbols (Alligood & Tomey, 2009).

A primary concept in the theory of transcultural nursing is that of cultural diversity, which are the variations observed between cultures. The nurse who is capable of recognizing the variations among cultures can avoid inadvertently stereotyping patients and thus assuming that all patients will respond to a "generic" plan for nursing care in the same manner. Similarly, another important concept of the theory is that of cultural universality, meaning the similarities that exist in various cultures when they are scrutinized. The nurse who recognizes such similarities is capable of recognizing the impact that health, healthy practices, and instruction on the maintenance of wellness have on the general well-being of entire cultural groups (Alligood & Tomey, 2009).

The goal of the theory of transcultural nursing is to plan culturally congruent nursing care based on knowledge that has been culturally defined. Leininger encouraged the registered nurse to be creative in attempts to discover the cultural aspects of the needs of patients and then use these discoveries in designing culturally congruent nursing care. She believed caring was the essence of nursing, and such caring encompassed nursing practice that respects the patient's culture. When culturally congruent care is implemented appropriately, the outcome will be a high level of health and well-being for the patient (Chitty & Black, 2010).

Several concepts are considered to be unique to Leininger's theory:

- **Ethnicity** is the awareness of belonging to a specific group.
- **Acculturation** means members of a minority group usually assume the beliefs, practices, and values of the dominant cultural group in the society so that a blending of the cultural group occurs.
- **Cultural awareness** occurs when the nurse examines their own background to assist in recognizing the existence of biases, prejudices, and assumptions that are present about other people.
- **Culturally congruent care** is nursing care that respects the patient's values and life patterns (McElwen & Wills, 2018).

Table 2.11 highlights the concepts that are unique to Leininger's theory of nursing.

TABLE 2.11. Basic Concepts of Leininger's Theory of Nursing

CONCEPT	DESCRIPTION
ethnicity	awareness of belonging to a specific group
acculturation	members of a minority group assume beliefs, practices, and values of the dominant cultural group so that a blending of the cultural group occurs
cultural awareness	nurse examines personal background to assist in recognizing existence of biases, prejudices, and assumptions
culturally congruent care	nursing care respects patient's values and life patterns

Source: McElwen, M., & Wills, E. (2018). Theoretical basis for nursing *(5th ed.). Lippincott, Williams, and Wilkins.*

Summary of Key Points in Chapter

Some of the most influential nursing theorists' contributions to nursing were discussed in this chapter, with each theorist's major assumptions, unique concepts, and developed proposals described. The following theorists were discussed:

- Virginia Henderson
- Imogene King

- Madeleine Leininger
- Betty Neuman
- Florence Nightingale
- Dorothea Orem
- Ida Jean Orlando
- Hildegard Peplau
- Martha Rogers
- Sister Callista Roy

This chapter includes tables outlining the key points of the theories developed by each of the respective theorists listed above.

Conclusion

The registered nurse will develop a more in-depth understanding of the theorists and their contribution to nursing as they progress through the process of becoming a nurse leader. This was by no means intended to be an exhaustive discussion of every prominent nursing theorist but will hopefully pique the interest of the new registered nurse to do additional research. Many of the reviewed theorists have models they developed that use their specific concepts.

The process of developing into a nurse leader includes acquiring the knowledge needed to guide change when it must occur in an organization, and many of the theories addressed here could prove foundational to such a process. The details of the change process itself and how the registered nurse can successfully function as a change agent are discussed in the next chapter.

Critical Thinking Questions

1. Consider Virginia Henderson's theory of nursing.
   a. Discuss the major assumptions of this theory.

b. Does this theory include a relationship to health? If so, describe the relationship.

c. Does this theory include a relationship to the nursing process? If so, describe the relationship.

d. Does this theory include a relationship to the environment? If so, describe the relationship.

2. Consider Imogene King's theory of nursing.

   a. Discuss the major assumptions of this theory.

b. Does this theory include a relationship to health? If so, describe the relationship.

c. Does this theory include a relationship to the nursing process? If so, describe the relationship.

d. Does this theory include a relationship to the environment? If so, describe the relationship.

3. Consider Madeleine Leininger's theory of nursing.

a. Discuss the major assumptions of this theory.

b. Does this theory include a relationship to health? If so, describe the relationship.

c. Does this theory include a relationship to the nursing process? If so, describe the relationship.

d. Does this theory include a relationship to the environment? If so, describe the relationship.

4. Consider Betty Neuman's theory of nursing.

   a. Discuss the major assumptions of this theory.

   b. Does this theory include a relationship to health? If so, describe the relationship.

   c. Does this theory include a relationship to the nursing process? If so, describe the relationship.

   d. Does this theory include a relationship to the environment? If so, describe the relationship.

5. Consider Florence Nightingale's theory of nursing.

   a. Discuss the major assumptions of this theory.

b. Does this theory include a relationship to health? If so, describe the relationship.

c. Does this theory include a relationship to the nursing process? If so, describe the relationship.

d. Does this theory include a relationship to the environment? If so, describe the relationship.

6. Consider Dorothea Orem's theory of nursing.

a. Discuss the major assumptions of this theory.

b. Does this theory include a relationship to health? If so, describe the relationship.

c. Does this theory include a relationship to the nursing process? If so, describe the relationship.

d. Does this theory include a relationship to the environment? If so, describe the relationship.

7. Consider Ida Orlando's theory of nursing.

   a. Discuss the major assumptions of this theory.

   b. Does this theory include a relationship to health? If so, describe the relationship.

   c. Does this theory include a relationship to the nursing process? If so, describe the relationship.

   d. Does this theory include a relationship to the environment? If so, describe the relationship.

8. Consider Hildegard Peplau's theory of nursing.

   a. Discuss the major assumptions of this theory.

   b. Does this theory include a relationship to health? If so, describe the relationship.

   c. Does this theory include a relationship to the nursing process? If so, describe the relationship.

   d. Does this theory include a relationship to the environment? If so, describe the relationship.

9. Consider Martha Rogers' theory of nursing.

   a. Discuss the major assumptions of this theory.

b. Does this theory include a relationship to health? If so, describe the relationship.

c. Does this theory include a relationship to the nursing process? If so, describe the relationship.

d. Does this theory include a relationship to the environment? If so, describe the relationship.

10. Consider Sister Callista Roy's theory of nursing.

a. Discuss the major assumptions of this theory.

b. Does this theory include a relationship to health? If so, describe the relationship.

c. Does this theory include a relationship to the nursing process? If so, describe the relationship.

d. Does this theory include a relationship to the environment? If so, describe the relationship.

▶ Scenarios

1. Discuss a situation in your current job in which you envision yourself using Virginia Henderson's theory of nursing in patient care.

   a. Has there ever been a time in your current job when you now realize Henderson's theory of nursing could have been used to explain a situation? If so, describe it in detail.

   b. If this theory could not have been used, is there a different theory of nursing that could have been useful at the time?

2. Discuss a situation in your current job when you can envision yourself using Imogene King's theory of nursing in patient care.

    a. Has there ever been a time in your current job when you now realize King's theory of nursing could have been used to explain a situation? If so, describe it in detail.

    b. If this theory could not have been used, is there a different theory of nursing that could have been useful at the time?

3. Discuss a situation in your current job in which you envision yourself using Madeleine Leininger's theory of nursing in patient care.

a. Has there ever been a time in your current job when you now realize Leininger's theory of nursing could have been used to explain a situation? If so, describe it in detail.

b. If this theory could not have been used, is there a different theory of nursing that could have been useful at the time?

4. Discuss a situation in your current job when you can envision yourself using Betty Neuman's theory of nursing in patient care.

   a. Has there ever been a time in your current job when you now realize Neuman's theory of nursing could have been used to explain a situation? If so, describe it in detail.

   b. If this theory could not have been used, is there a different theory of nursing that could have been useful at the time?

5. Discuss a situation in your current job in which you envision yourself using Florence Nightingale's theory of nursing in patient care.

   a. Has there ever been a time in your current job when you now realize Nightingale's theory of nursing could have been used to explain a situation? If so, describe it in detail.

   b. If this theory could not have been used, is there a different theory of nursing that could have been useful at the time?

6. Discuss a situation in your current job in which you envision yourself using Dorothea Orem's theory of nursing in patient care.

a. Has there ever been a time in your current job when you now realize Orem's theory of nursing could have been used to explain a situation? If so, describe it in detail.

b. If this theory could not have been used, is there a different theory of nursing that could have been useful at the time?

7. Discuss a situation in your current job when you can envision yourself using Ida Orlando's theory of nursing in patient care.

a. Has there ever been a time in your current job when you now realize Orlando's theory of nursing could have been used to explain a situation? If so, describe it in detail.

b. If this theory could not have been used, is there a different theory of nursing that could have been useful at the time?

8. Discuss a situation in your current job in which you envision yourself using Hildegard Peplau's theory of nursing in patient care.

    a. Has there ever been a time in your current job when you now realize Peplau's theory of nursing could have been used to explain a situation? If so, describe it in detail.

    b. If this theory could not have been used, is there a different theory of nursing that could have been useful at the time?

9. Discuss a situation in your current job when you can envision yourself using Martha Rogers' theory of nursing in patient care.

    a. Has there ever been a time in your current job when you now realize Rogers' theory of nursing could have been used to explain a situation? If so, describe it in detail.

b. If this theory could not have been used, is there a different theory of nursing that could have been useful at the time?

10. Discuss a situation in your current job in which you can envision yourself using Sister Callista Roy's theory of nursing in patient care.

    a. Has there ever been a time in your current job when you now realize Roy's theory of nursing could have been used to explain a situation? If so, describe it in detail.

    b. If this theory could not have been used, is there a different theory of nursing that could have been useful at the time?

11. Select one of the nursing theories discussed in this chapter that appeals to you the most. Discuss why this particular theory appeals to you and how you will apply it in your daily nursing practice.

12. Compare and contrast Nightingale's theory of nursing with Orem's theory of nursing.

13. Compare and contrast King's theory of nursing with Neuman's theory of nursing.

14. Compare and contrast Rogers' theory of nursing with Roy's theory of nursing.

15. Compare and contrast Orlando's theory of nursing with Peplau's theory of nursing.

NCLEX-Style Review Questions

1. Select the nursing theory that contains the following concepts:
   a. ____ nursing, individual, health, environment
   b. ____ ethnicity, acculturation, cultural awareness, culturally congruent care
   c. ____ human being, intrapersonal stressors, interpersonal stressors, extrapersonal stressors
   d. ____ distress, nursing role, nursing actions, outcome, nursing, outcome, nursing client
   e. ____ stranger, teacher, resource person, counselor, surrogate, leader
   f. ____ unitary human being, energy field, scope of nursing, health
   g. ____ adaptation, focal stimuli, contextual stimuli, residual stimuli

   Roy's theory
   Rogers' theory
   Leininger's theory
   Peplau's theory
   Henderson's theory
   Orem's theory
   Orlando's theory
   Neuman's theory

2. Documentation of the interaction that occurs between concepts and the patterns that result from that interaction form a:
   a. proposition
   b. process
   c. model
   d. conceptual framework

3. Statements that explain relationships between the concepts used in a certain theory form a:
   a. proposition
   b. process
   c. model
   d. conceptual framework

4. A series of actions, proposed changes, or functions that are implemented to bring about a specific result forms a:
   a. proposition
   b. process
   c. model
   d. conceptual framework

5. Functions that are basic needs of the individual according to Henderson's theory include:
   a. financial stability
   b. cultural competence
   c. verbalizing thoughts
   d. participating in recreation

6. Madeleine Leininger's theory of nursing is based on the science of:
   a. psychology
   b. sociology
   c. anthropology
   d. pathophysiology

7. According to Leininger's theory, the belief that members of a minority group usually assume the beliefs, practices, and values of the dominant cultural group in the society so that a blending of the cultural group occurs is known as:
   a. ethnicity
   b. acculturation
   c. cultural awareness
   d. culturally congruent care

8. According to Leininger's theory, the awareness of belonging to a specific group is known as:
   a. ethnicity
   b. acculturation
   c. cultural awareness
   d. culturally congruent care

9. According to Leininger's theory, _______________ exists when the nurse examines their own background to assist in recognizing the existence of biases, prejudices, and assumptions that are present about other people.
   a. ethnicity
   b. acculturation
   c. cultural awareness
   d. culturally congruent care

10. Which one of the subtheories that compose Orem's theory of nursing explained why individuals can be helped through nursing?
   a. theory of self-care
   b. theory of self-care deficit
   c. theory of nursing systems
   d. theory of diagnostic operations

11. Which one of the subtheories that compose Orem's theory of nursing described why the individual will choose to care for themselves?
   a. theory of self-care
   b. theory of self-care deficit
   c. theory of nursing systems
   d. theory of diagnostic operations

12. Which one of the subtheories that compose Orem's theory of nursing proposed relationships that must be both developed and maintained in order for nursing to be implemented?
   a. theory of self-care
   b. theory of self-care deficit
   c. theory of nursing systems
   d. theory of diagnostic operations

13. Which one of the subtheories that compose Orem's theory of nursing described how care provided to the individual through nursing can be beneficial?
   a. theory of self-care
   b. theory of self-care deficit
   c. theory of nursing systems
   d. theory of diagnostic operations

14. Which one of the subtheories that compose Orem's theory of nursing attempted to explain the nature of the relationships that must be both developed and maintained in order for nursing to be implemented?
   a. theory of self-care
   b. theory of self-care deficit
   c. theory of nursing systems

15. The home health nurse is working with a population of patients who have cultural beliefs that are different from her own. The nursing theory that would be most useful to her would be:
    a. Orem's theory
    b. Peplau's theory
    c. Leininger's theory
    d. Roy's theory

16. The nurse is working with a patient who is undergoing chemotherapy to treat cancer. To lessen the side effects of the chemotherapy that the patient is experiencing, the nurse attempts to use scientific problem-solving methods to make decisions. This most closely aligns with which one of Watson's carative factors?
    a. balance
    b. deepen
    c. inspire
    d. minister

▸ Note Taker

I. Virginia Henderson's theory of nursing

   A. Needs of the individual

   B. Primary concepts of the theory

C. Imogene King's theory of nursing

D. Steps in the communication process

E. Primary concepts of the theory

II. Madeleine Leininger's theory of nursing

A. Transcultural nursing

B. Primary concepts of the theory

III. Betty Neuman's theory of nursing

A. Stressors

B. Client system

C. Primary concepts of the theory

IV. Florence Nightingale's theory of nursing

A. Expectations of nurses

B. Primary concepts of the theory

V. Dorothea Orem's theory of nursing

A. Theory of self-care

B. Theory of self-care deficit

C. Theory of nursing systems

D. Primary concepts of the theory

VI. Ida Orlando's theory of nursing

A. Dimensions to the theory

B. Primary concepts of the theory

VII. Hildegard Peplau's theory of nursing

A. Phases of the nurse-patient relationship

B. Primary concepts of the theory

VIII. Martha Rogers's theory of nursing

A. Unitary human being

B. Primary concepts of the theory

IX. Sister Callista Roy's theory of nursing

A. Human adaptive behavior

B. Stages of the nursing process

C. Primary concepts of the theory

References

Alligood, M., & Tomey, A. (2009). *Nursing theory: Utilization and application* (4th ed.). Elsevier.

Chinn, P., & Kramer, M. (2010). *Integrated theory and knowledge development in nursing.* Elsevier.

Chitty, K., & Black, B. (2010). *Professional nursing: Concepts and challenges* (6th ed.). Elsevier.

McElwen, M., & Wills, E. (2018). *Theoretical basis for nursing* (5th ed.). Lippincott, Williams, and Wilkins.

McKenna, H. (2002). *Nursing theories and models.* Routledge.

Parker, M., & Smith, M. (2010). *Nursing theories and nursing practice* (3rd ed.) F. A. Davis.

Psych-Mental Health Hub. (n.d.). *Jean Watson theory of human science and human caring.* https://pmhealthnp.com/jean-watson-theory-of-human-science-and-human-caring/

Reed, P., & Shearer, N. (2011). *Perspectives on nursing theory.* Lippincott, Williams, and Wilkins.

Tomey, A., & Alligood, M. (2010). *Nursing theorists and their work* (7th ed.). Elsevier.

CHAPTER 3

Nursing Licensure

KEY TERMS

licensure
licensure by examination
regulation
Nurse Practice Act
Nurse Licensure Compact
discipline of a license

CHAPTER OBJECTIVES

Upon completion of the chapter, you will be able to:

1. Discuss the necessity of licensure to ensure practice as a registered nurse
2. Describe the purpose for a Nurse Practice Act in each state and territory
3. Describe the requirements for licensure by examination as a registered nurse
4. Discuss the Nurse Licensure Compact and identify whether your home state is a member of the compact
5. Discuss the different types of disciplinary cases that are reviewed by boards of nursing

A significant aspect of nursing as a profession is the licensure of its members to practice. Licensure is necessary to protect the health, safety, and welfare of the public since nursing is a profession that can produce harm if practiced incorrectly. Nursing is a profession that requires specialized knowledge, specific skills, and the ability to utilize both critical thinking and problem solving effectively. Furthermore, nurses are becoming more mobile than ever before as state boards of nursing move toward compact nursing licensure that allows nurses to practice in multiple states. These areas contribute to the need to regulate the profession through licensure to protect the public from individuals who are either unprepared or incompetent to practice nursing (Russell, 2012). Fowler (2015) noted that nursing as a helping profession has a relationship—literally a "social contract"—with society, and because of this, both parties in the contract are allowed to have expectations. Nursing meets the societal needs for health, and society in turn assists nursing to utilize political and legislative action that will support nursing education, research, and practice.

Introduction to the Nursing Licensure Process

Nursing is considered to be a regulated profession, meaning that each state's legislative body establishes practice law and then assigns authority to implement the law to an entity such as a State Board of Nursing. The first state to require licensure of nurses was North Carolina in 1903 (Michaels, 2021). Today boards of nursing are typically composed of registered nurses, license practical nurses, advanced practice nurses, and consumer. What are the functions of a state board of nursing? According to the National Council of State Boards of Nursing (2018), a board of nursing can:

- **Evaluate licensure applications:** The board evaluates each application to determine if applicants possess appropriate educational credentials, have successfully passed the NCLEX-RN licensure exam, and have successfully completed the background check.
- **Issue licenses:** The board issues nursing licenses and maintains a list of licensed nurses. The lists are available to the public and to health care providers.
- **Renew licenses:** Each board determines specific renewal requirements, but in general, in order to renew a license, a nurse must fulfill a requirement for a certain number of continuing education units and must also be in good standing.
- **Take disciplinary action:** If a nurse is found to violate a law or a complaint is brought against the nurse by a member of the public, the board of nursing will initiate an investigation and may choose to take disciplinary action against the nurse's license.

Boards of nursing do not determine the curricula for nursing programs.

The professional Nurse Practice Act will set the standard for licensure as a nurse in each state. All 50 states as well as the District of Columbia and the U.S. territories have nurse practice acts that have been established by their legislatures to regulate nursing in each area. Nurse Practice Acts are important because they are designed to meet the following objectives:

- Define the practice of professional nursing in that state or territory
- Establish the minimum educational qualification for licensure
- Determine other requirements for licensure
- Establish the legal titles and abbreviations that may be used by the professional nurse
- Provide a process for the disciplinary action of licensed professional nurses when needed (Black, 2014)

The process of nursing licensure is also important because it establishes that the title of "nurse" can only be used by individuals who have met the legal and educational standards. Nurse Practice Acts will usually include a statement protecting the titles of registered nurse (RN) and licensed practical nurse (LPN) from use by unauthorized individuals. The Nurse Practice Act will also include information on the requirements for examination for licensure as RNs and LPN. Each state and territory's requirements for licensure by examination typically will consist of the following:

- Completion of application and payment of fee
- Graduation from an approved program that meets the criteria established by the state
- Passage of the National Council Licensure Examination (NCLEX) professional licensure examination
- Attesting to no reported substance abuse within the past five years
- Verifying that no actions were taken or initiated against any type of professional license, registration, or certification

- Attesting to reported acts or omissions that would be grounds for disciplinary action as specified in the state's Nurse Practice Act
- Criminal background check (Russell, 2012)

Because of the mobility of modern society, the National Council of State Boards of Nursing developed the Nurse Licensure Compact in 2000. This model of licensure allows an RN to have a licensure in the state of residency while practicing nursing in other compact member states without an additional license in the state of employment. The nurse will be subject to the Nurse Practice Act in the state where the nurse is practicing. This model of licensure should provide for improved public protection through improved tracking of nurses who have sustained discipline of their licenses (Black, 2014). It is important to note that not all states have opted to become a compact state.

Sustaining Discipline of a Nursing License

A nurse can sustain discipline of a license if the person does not provide a satisfactory level of care and a complaint is lodged with a board of nursing. Because of the authority that it has from the Nurse Practice Act, the board of nursing has the responsibility to review all complaints made against nurses. If there is sufficient evidence that the nurse violated state laws or regulations, the board of nursing will take formal disciplinary action (Russell, 2012).

Following are the categories of disciplinary cases that are reviewed by boards of nursing:

- Practice-related: This means there has been a breach in the standard of nursing care provided to a patient. Examples include a failure to assess a change in the patient's condition, failure to implement an ordered intervention, failure to document nursing care provided, and failure to follow the proper procedure for drug administration.
- Drug-related: This means that nurses have misused controlled substances. Examples include misappropriating patient medications, failing to document medication administration, being impaired as a nurse through medication usage, and using unauthorized prescriptions to attempt to obtain medications.
- Boundary violations: This means that the nurse forms a nontherapeutic relationship with a patient that leads to the nurse deriving a benefit at the expense of the patient. Examples include establishing a personal relationship with a current or former patient for personal gratification and sharing personal information with patients to obtain money or gifts.
- Sexual misconduct: This means that the patient experiences physician or sexual abuse from a nurse. The abuse may be a boundary violation extending from a nontherapeutic nurse-patient relationship.
- Abuse: This means mistreatment of a patient that results in physical, emotional, or mental harm.
- Fraud: This means that the nurse misrepresents the truth for some type of gain. Examples include reporting credentials that were not actually obtained, claiming hours that were not actually worked, falsely documenting care that could result in payments, and submitting inaccurate billing records.

- Positive criminal background check: This means that licensure consequences may occur based on the degree and severity of the nurse's past criminal conduct and the risk to patients from a future lapse in the nurse's judgment (National Council of State Boards of Nursing, 2021; see Table 3.1).

TABLE 3.1. Categories of Discipline for a Nursing License

TYPE OF DISCIPLINE	DESCRIPTION	EXAMPLES
Practice-related	There has been a breach in the standard of nursing care provided to a patient.	1. Failure to assess a change in the patient's condition 2. Failure to implement an ordered intervention 3. Failure to document nursing care provided 4. Failure to follow the proper procedure for drug administration
Drug-related	Nurses have misused controlled substances.	1. Misappropriating patient medications 2. Failing to document medication administration 3. Being impaired as a nurse through medication usage 4. Using unauthorized prescriptions to attempt to obtain medications
Boundary violations	The nurse forms a nontherapeutic relationship with a patient that leads to the nurse deriving a benefit at the expense of the patient.	a. Establishing a personal relationship with a current or former patient for personal gratification b. Sharing personal information with patients to obtain money or gifts
Sexual misconduct	The patient experiences physical or sexual abuse from a nurse.	The abuse may be a boundary violation extending from a nontherapeutic nurse-patient relationship.
Abuse	This type of abuse occurs when there is mistreatment of a patient that results in physical, emotional, or mental harm.	There is a clear relationship between the patient's treatment and the resulting harm.

TYPE OF DISCIPLINE	DESCRIPTION	EXAMPLES
Fraud	The nurse misrepresents the truth for some type of gain.	1. Reporting credentials that were not actually obtained 2. Claiming hours that were not actually worked 3. Falsely documenting that could result in payments 4. Submitting inaccurate billing records
Positive criminal background check	Licensure consequences may occur based on the degree and severity of the nurse's past criminal conduct and the risk to patients from a future lapse in the nurse's judgment.	

It is important that all nurses recognize how discipline of the license can occur so that such violations can be avoided. Become familiar with your state's Nurse Practice Act as well as the website for the Board of Nursing.

▸ Summary of Key Points in Chapter

This chapter discussed the necessity of licensure for the registered nurse to practice in today's world. Important concepts discussed are:

- Nursing as a regulated profession
- The purposes of Nurse Practice Acts
- Requirements for licensure by examination
- Nurse Licensure Compact
- Types of discipline of a nursing license:
- Practice-related
- Drug-related
- Boundary violation
- Sexual misconduct
- Abuse

▸ Conclusion

Nursing as a regulated profession has progressed significantly from the initial requirement for licensure for nurses in North Carolina in 1903 until the initiation of the modern compact license that exists today. Will licensure requirements change as nurses struggle to cope with the staffing challenges posed by disasters such as the COVID-19 pandemic? The National Council of State Boards of Nurses released a statement in 2021 regarding its position on emergency action by states severely affected by a public health disaster whose governors have declared a state of emergency (2021).

As nursing continues to be buffeted by these challenges, part of its coping response will be to determine the proper way to respond to the resulting legal and ethical questions that will also emerge. Legal and ethical aspects of nursing will be discussed in the subsequent chapters.

▶ Critical Thinking Questions

1. Go to the National Council of State Boards of Nursing website (https://www.ncsbn.org/npa.htm) and locate the Nurse Practice Act for your home state. Review the purposes of the Nurse Practice Act. Is there one that you believe is more important than the others? Explain your answer.

2. Go to the section of the National Council of State Boards of Nursing website that pertains to each state's board of nursing (https://www.ncsbn.org/contact-bon.htm) and locate the board of nursing for your home state. Review your state's requirements for licensure as a nurse by examination.

    a. Is there one of the requirements that you believe is more important than the others? Explain your answer.

    b. Is there one of the requirements that you believe needs to be revised or is outdated? Explain your answer.

c. A registered nurse works for a home health agency. One of his patients is Mr. Smith, a 75-year-old cancer patient whose caregiver is his granddaughter Julie. The nurse begins dating Julie. Do you think that the nurse risks discipline of his license? Explain your answer.

3. A registered nurse is preparing her resume, hoping for a new position in an intensive care unit. She has an associate degree in nursing and lacks only one-quarter completion of a degree in business. She will be applying for a position as the assistant nurse manager and wonders if a degree in business would give her an advantage over other applicants. On her resume, she indicates that she has already completed the degree in business. Do you think that the nurse risks discipline of her license? Explain your answer.

▶ Scenarios

1. Go to the section of the National Council of State Boards of Nursing website that pertains to each state's board of nursing (https://www.ncsbn.org/contact-bon.htm) and locate the board of nursing for your home state. Review your state's requirements for licensure as a nurse by examination. You have been appointed to a committee that has been charged with reviewing the requirements and developing new ones where needed. Develop the new list of revised requirements and be able to explain why each one was revised, rejected, or newly written.

2. You are working as a registered nurse on a medical-surgical floor. You are working today with your friend Sue on the 7 a.m.–7 p.m. shift. Sue comes to find you during the shift to tell you that she has been notified that a complaint has been made by someone in the public about the care that she delivered to a patient who died last week. The complaint stated that Sue administered the wrong amount of a cardiac medication to the patient and that this resulted in cardiac arrest. Sue is pale and tells you in a whisper, "It's true; I did it, but I didn't think that anybody knew about it!"

    a. Which types of discipline of her license is Sue at risk to sustain?

    b. What should Sue have done once she recognized that she administered too much of the medication? To answer this, go to the section of the National Council of State Boards of Nursing website that pertains to each state's Board of Nursing (https://www.ncsbn.org/contact-bon.htm) and locate the board of nursing for your home state. Determine the board of nursing's requirements for reporting such errors.

    c. What do you view as your responsibility in Sue's case? Explain your answer.

NCLEX-Style Review Questions

1. You are reviewing your state's Nurse Practice Act. You recognize that the purposes of the Nurse Practice Act include all of the following (*select all that apply*):
   a. Establish the legal titles and abbreviations that may be used by the professional nurse.
   b. Establish the minimum educational qualification for licensure.
   c. Define the practice of professional nursing that applies nationwide.
   d. Provide a process for the disciplinary action of licensed professional nurses when needed.
   e. Discipline nurses' licenses as needed.

2. Examples of practice-related actions that could result in discipline include all of the following: (*select all that apply*)
   a. Failing to document medication administration
   b. Failing to assess a change in the patient's condition
   c. Failing to implement an ordered intervention
   d. Failing to document nursing care provided
   e. Failing to follow the proper procedure for drug administration

3. The nurse tells her patient that the nurse's child needs expensive surgery. The patient offers her the money for the surgery, and the patient accepts it. The nurse is at risk for which type of discipline on her license?
   a. Fraud
   b. Abuse
   c. Boundary violation
   d. Practice-Related

4. The nurse fails to document an administered medication. The nurse is at risk for which type of discipline on her license?
   a. Boundary violation
   b. Drug-related
   c. Practice-related
   d. Fraud

5. Examples of drug-related actions that could result in discipline include all of the following: (*select all that apply*)
   a. Misappropriating patient medications
   b. Forming a nontherapeutic relationship with the patient
   c. Failing to document medication administration
   d. Being impaired as a nurse through medication usage
   e. Using unauthorized prescriptions to attempt to obtain medications

▶ Case Study

Your friend Jordan just graduated from an associate degree nursing program and is preparing to seek licensure as a registered nurse. He tells you that he is concerned about his ability to successfully complete the licensure process because he is afraid that he will fail the background check. When you question him further, he relates that he had a drug charge when he was 17 but assumed that his record was clear because his attorney told him that he had youthful offender status in his home state.

1. Jordan is at risk for disciplinary action from the board of nursing based on (*select all that apply*):
   a. Practice-related violation
   b. Drug-related violation
   c. Breach in the standard of nursing care
   d. Sexual misconduct violation
   e. Misuse of controlled substances
   f. Nontherapeutic relationship with a patient
   g. Positive criminal background check
   h. Boundary violation
   i. Risk to patients from future lapse in judgment
   j. Misrepresenting the truth for gain
2. To successfully attain licensure, Jordan will need to successfully (*select all that apply*):
   a. Complete application and pay fee
   b. Graduate from an approved program
   c. Pass NCLEX
   d. Attest to no reported substance abuse within the past 10 years
   e. Verify that no actions were taken against any type of professional license
   f. Attest to reported acts that would be grounds for disciplinary action
   g. Have a criminal background check (Russell, 2012)
3. What should you advise Jordan to do?

▶ Concept Map

Develop a concept map based on Jordan's situation.

▶ Note Taker

I. Necessity of licensure

II. Purposes of the Nurse Practice Act

A. Define the practice of professional nursing in that state or territory.

B. Establish the minimum educational qualification for licensure.

C. Determine other requirements for licensure.

D. Establish the legal titles and abbreviations that may be used by the professional nurse.

E. Provide a process for the disciplinary action of licensed professional nurses when needed.

III. Requirements for licensure by examination

A. Completion of application and payment of fee

B. Graduation from an approved program that meets the criteria established by the state

C. Passage of the NCLEX professional licensure examination

D. Attesting to no reported substance abuse within the past five years

E. Verifying that no actions were taken or initiated against any type of professional license, registration, or certification

F. Attesting to reported acts or omissions that would be grounds for disciplinary action as specified in the state's Nurse Practice Act

G. Criminal background check

IV. Nurse Licensure Compact

V. Categories of discipline of nursing license

A. Practice-related

B. Drug-related

C. Boundary violations

D. Sexual misconduct

E. Abuse

F. Fraud

G. Positive criminal background check

References

Black, B. P. (2014). *Professional nursing: Concepts and challenges* (7th ed.). Elsevier.

Fowler, M. (2015). *Guide to nursing's social policy statement: Understanding the profession from social contract to social covenant*. American Nurses Association.

Michaels, D. (2021, February 4). *Nurse licensure and registration*. https://www.americannursinghistory.org/nursinglicensure-and-registration

National Council of State Boards of Nursing. (2018). *What every nurse needs to know about state and territorial boards of nursing*. https://www.ncsbn.org/What_Every_Nurse_Needs_to_Know.pdf

National Council of State Boards of Nursing. (2021). *Emergency response by state and nurse*. https://www.ncsbn.org/14508.htm.

National Council of State Boards of Nursing. (2021). *Initial review of complaint*. https://www.ncsbn.org/1616.htm#6038.

Russell, K. (2012). Nurse practice acts guide and govern nursing practice. *Journal of Nursing Regulation, 3*(3), 36–42.

PART II

Transition Into the Professional Nurse Role

CHAPTER

4

Ethical Issues in Nursing

CHAPTER OBJECTIVES

Upon completion of the chapter, you will be able to:

1. Define the primary ethical principles
2. Discuss the importance of the American Nurses' Association's code of ethics
3. Recognize the characteristics of an ethical dilemma
4. Discuss the stages of the ethical decision-making process
5. Describe the difference between an ethical dilemma and moral distress

KEY TERMS

American Nurses Association code of ethics
autonomy
beneficence
confidentiality
ethical dilemma
euthanasia
fidelity
futile care
justice
malpractice
morals
moral courage
moral distress
negligence
nonmaleficence
Nurse Practice Act
privacy
role conflict
values
veracity

Ethical issues in the nursing profession can frequently be intertwined with legal issues as well. Legal issues will be addressed in the next chapter. *Ethics in nursing* is a somewhat nebulous term but essentially refers to morals and values used when health care professionals make life-and-death decisions involving patients and their care. It is the system of beliefs about what makes moral conduct. The nurse who acts in an ethical manner accepts responsibility and accountability for actions. Values, morals, and ethics can have overlapping areas. ***Values*** are considered to be the ideals, beliefs, and behavior patterns that you choose. They are learned behaviors that are usually influenced by your culture, ethnicity, level of education, and various life experiences. ***Morals***, in comparison, are considered to be a standard conduct. They tend to represent the ideal in human behavior and serve as a guideline in our relationships with others.

Health care professionals, and nurses in particular, frequently are faced with an ethical dilemma—a situation in which there seem to be a conflict between two separate ethical duties. The nurse will be uncertain of the correct moral action (Huber, 2010). The registered nurse (RN) faced with the existence of an ethical dilemma should first ensure that the nurse has a sufficient understanding of important ethical principles:

Autonomy: This is the patient's right to make their own decisions.

Beneficence: This means the nurse wants to do good for the patient and balances the potential benefit to the patient with the potential risk.

Nonmaleficence: This means avoiding doing harm to the patient.

Justice: This equates to providing fair and equal treatment to all patients and to ensuring that benefits, risks, and costs are equally distributed so that no one group or individual bears the burden exclusively.

Fidelity: This pertains to being loyal to commitments that have been made and accountable for responsibilities.

Veracity: This pertains to avoiding misleading patients.

Confidentiality: This pertains to the amount of information that can be disclosed about a patient without their consent.

Privacy: This pertains to limiting the amount of information to disclose about oneself.

These principles pertaining to ethics must be well understood by the RN before an ethical dilemma develops so that valuable time is not spent in lengthy deliberation (Huber, 2010).

ANA Code of Ethics

In addition to a clear understanding of the principles that form the foundation of nursing ethics, the RN should also adhere to the **American Nurses Association's** (ANA) **code of ethics**, a document containing the ethical obligations and duties of the nurse. The code does not provide specific answers for every ethical issue that could be faced by a nurse but instead provides general principles used to make decisions when the nurse is confronted with various types of ethical decisions. However, there are several areas of ethical uncertainty in which the ANA code of ethics does provide more specific guidance to the RN (Huber, 2010):

- Patient's right to die
- Use of incentives to decrease spending in health care
- Confronted with questionable or impaired practice of a colleague
- Patient whose medical needs exceed the nurse's knowledge base and skill set
- Organization creating barriers to ethical practice

Ethical Decision-Making

How should the RN go about resolving an ethical dilemma when there seems to be a conflict between the professional duty owed to the patient, the rights of the patient, and possibly even the religious beliefs of the nurse? The basic problem-solving process can be modified to fit this situation (Huber, 2010):

- Define the problem by breaking it down into manageable terms. It may be easier to make a decision if the problem is broken down into a series of smaller problems that may be more easily solved.
- Determine the alternatives that are not only available but also options that are viable. If an alternative would only be feasible if there were additional equipment, personnel, and funding, it is not a true alternative.

- Evaluate all alternative courses of action, determining how easily each would be implemented, the resources that would be required, the benefits to all persons involved, and the drawbacks.
- Choose the best course of action based on weighing the benefits and the drawbacks.
- Implement the selected course of action, documenting every step of the process of implementation.
- Evaluate the results of the implementation process, monitoring it closely to provide guidance in the event that such an ethical dilemma occurs again.

The ethical decision-making process is summarized below.

Define the problem by breaking it down into manageable terms.

Determine the alternatives that are not only available but are truly options that are viable.

Evaluate all alternative courses of action.

- How easily will each be implemented?
- What are the resources that would be required?
- What are the benefits to all persons involved?
- What are the drawbacks?

Choose the best course of action based on weighing the benefits and the drawbacks.

Implement the selected course of action, documenting every step of the process of implementation.

Evaluate the results of the implementation process

FIGURE 4.1. Ethical Decision-Making Process

Ethical Issues Related to Death and Dying

Multiple ethical dilemmas can emerge from the controversy that often surrounds the dying process and subsequent death. Frequently, nurses care for patients whose physicians have written "do not resuscitate" orders. These orders are enacted such that cardiopulmonary resuscitation is not used in the event the patient begins to exhibit signs that their physical condition is deteriorating. Such an order may be difficult for the nurse who believes that failing to resuscitate the patient is directly contributing to the patient's death and thus is in conflict with the nurse's duty to the patient (Rumbold, 1999).

For many RNs implementing such orders can create an ethical dilemma because of the nurse's concerns regarding euthanasia, the deliberate ending of life in the interest of ending the suffering of the patient. In addition, the nurse may have an ethical dilemma if called on to assist with a family's decision to withdraw life-sustaining treatment from a patient whose physical condition is deteriorating (Rumbold, 1999). This may conflict greatly with a nurse's commitment to sustain life as well as their religious beliefs regarding the sanctity of life.

Moral Distress

Ultimately, ethical dilemmas such as those just described can cause a nurse to experience ***moral distress***, which Gallagher (2010) defined as the nurse knowing the right decision to make in a specific circumstance but being prevented from making the right decision by constraints imposed by the facility. Moral distress can be caused by a combination of substandard health care delivery; **futile care**, meaning care that seems to provide no benefit for the patient; unsuccessful advocacy by the RN on the behalf of the patient; and the belief that the RN is raising the patient's and family's hope unrealistically.

In the hospital work environment, nurses report moral distress due to inadequate staffing as well as frequent confrontations with physicians. Research has shown that moral distress is associated with educational level and experience, suggesting nurses with advanced education and multiple years of experience tend to have higher levels of moral distress. It has been found to manifest itself physically in symptoms such as headaches, neck pain, and stomach problems and emotionally in the form of angry outbursts, feelings of guilt, frustration, low self-esteem, and isolation from loved ones. The main remedy for moral distress appears to be **moral courage**, which can be developed through the use of professional wisdom. The nurse who develops such wisdom typically is able to demonstrate the right response in the face of frightening encounters (Gallagher, 2010). Silverman et al. (2021) studied the moral distress that developed in nurses who were caring for patients during the COVID-19 pandemic and were faced with trying to provide superior care during staffing and equipment shortages and frequent patient fatalities.

An RN should develop ways of knowing when moral distress is developing. Pendry (2007) noted several situations in the modern health care environment that can lead to the development of moral distress:

1. **Role conflict:** This consists of the stress that develops when the expectations of two different areas of authority over a nurse are incongruent. For example, if the RN's hospital administration expects one thing from them and the physician who works closely with that nurse has a set of expectations that conflict with those of the hospital administration, role conflict results. Consequently, the RN will have more responsibility than authority and will lack the autonomy to accomplish what they believe needs to be done. The nurse will feel helpless and will believe that they are not able to provide high-quality health care to patients.
2. **Conflict between physicians and nurses:** Research has shown that the greatest conflict between physicians and nurses develops over end-of-life decision-making. Such conflicts can develop out of the multiple values that are involved, such as respect for human life as well as the patient's right to autonomy, the hierarchy of authority present in most health care organizations, the lack of resources to devote to the patient in the midst of the dying process, and the need for all parties involved in the end-of-life decision-making

process to have full communication with each other. Both physicians and nurses tend to express feelings of powerlessness in such a situation, with the physicians frequently expressing concern that selecting one patient to receive extended treatment might mean that another one receives a lesser degree of care, and nurses expressing concern that they are providing substandard care due to financial constraints. Research has shown that physicians typically feel the stress of making end-of-life decisions, whereas nurses feel the stress of implementing the mandates of a decision made by someone else.

3. **End-of-life care:** Nurses frequently report being extremely stressed when patients ask for assistance in dying, particularly when they have been experiencing prolonged suffering. Nurses often express great concern over unrelieved pain and distress of patients as well as being asked to withhold nutrition or administer larger than recommended doses of opioid analgesics in an attempt to accelerate the dying process.
4. **Conflict between critical care and futile care:** Critical care RNs are believed to experience particularly high levels of moral distress when called on to provide medically aggressive care to prolong life for a patient in a futile care situation, when it is clear that the patient is progressing into the dying process. It has been found that such a situation contributes significantly to the development of burnout in nurses, resulting in the RN experiencing emotional exhaustion, detachment, and a sense of lack of accomplishment. Moral distress can actually result from the critical care nurse's own expert judgment as a clinician because this sense will provide the nurse with a heightened perception of the inability to provide the patient with a prolonged quality of life.
5. **Managed care requirements:** RNs who function under a managed care system have expressed moral distress as a result of the frustration over feeling they are functioning primarily as an agent for the health plan rather than as an advocate for the patient. Many nurses have reported feeling the need to exaggerate aspects of the patient's illness or purposely inadequately document patient findings to provide greater resources to the patient under the managed care system. RNs functioning as case managers have also reported moral distress resulting from the frustration in dealing with insurance companies. The case manager may be faced with attempting to advocate for the patient while trying to balance the dictates of the insurance company regarding how extensive care can be and the expectations of family members.
6. **Conflict between new graduates' expectations and reality**: Research on the job satisfaction of new graduate nurses has shown that almost one-third of them report leaving their first nursing job within one year of being hired and more than half usually leave within two years. The new graduates who were surveyed reported they were greatly stressed by the acuity of the patients assigned to them, the nurse-to-patient ratios, their perceived inability to provide safe care, a lack of support and guidance, and a perception of having too much responsibility (Pendry, 2007).

▸ Summary of Key Points in Chapter

Although this chapter discussed ethical aspects of nursing, a wide variety of topics was presented. This included a discussion of the various ethical principles, the importance of the ANA code of ethics to the RN, and the process for resolving an ethical dilemma. Finally, the characteristics of moral distress were delineated, as were various factors that could contribute to development of such a situation.

▶ Conclusion

This chapter has shown multiple ethical issues at work in the modern health care environment, and most of them will, at some point, have an effect on the RN and the care that is delivered. It is the responsibility of the RN who is transitioning into the process of becoming a nurse leader to stay current with all available information on ethical issues that could affect not only personal practice but also the facility where that practice occurs. In addition, the RN nurse leader must maintain their status as a mentor and a role model in the health care community to recognize when other nurses are developing moral distress and circumvent this process when possible.

Ethical issues such as those connected with the end of life are particularly stressful to deal with for the RN and could potentially result in legal difficulties as well. Legal aspects of nursing are explored in the next chapter.

▶ Critical Thinking Questions

1. Consider a current or past work environment.
    a. Can you recall a time when you saw a nurse exhibit moral distress?
    b. Have you ever felt moral distress?
    c. Have you ever felt moral courage, or have you ever seen a nurse demonstrate it?

2. How would you explain the following ethical principles to a colleague?

   a. Autonomy

   b. Beneficence

   c. Nonmaleficence

   d. Justice

   e. Fidelity

   f. Veracity

   g. Confidentiality

h. Privacy

3. How would explain the ethical principles discussed in question 2 to a patient?

4. Compare and contrast the differences between an ethical dilemma and moral distress.

5. Compare and contrast morals, values, and ethics.

▶ Scenarios

1. You are the RN who is caring for a young adult patient who is on a ventilator due to COVID-19. The physician spoke with the patient's family today regarding removing the patient from the ventilator since the physician believes that nothing else can be done to improve the patient's chances of survival. You do not agree with the physician's assessment of the situation. Use the ethical decision-making process to resolve this ethical dilemma.

2. You are working with patients in a community clinic. One tells you, "I'm not going to get the COVID vaccine, and I'm not going to wear a mask either. My doctor told me that I don't have to and for me not to worry about it." Use the ethical decision-making process to resolve this ethical dilemma.

▶ NCLEX-Style Review Questions

1. The RN experiences frustration because the nurse reports knowing the right decision to make when caring for dying patients but is prevented from making the right decision by the hospital's policies. This is most likely to be:
   a. Role conflict
   b. Futile care
   c. Moral distress
   d. Moral courage

2. The unit manager finds the new graduate RN weeping in the break room. The RN tells the unit manager, "I tried so hard to get the doctor to increase Mrs. Jones' pain medication, and now it doesn't help her at all!" The RN is experiencing:
   a. Role conflict
   b. Futile care
   c. Moral distress
   d. Moral courage

3. The RN experiences stress because the physician has written orders for some expensive supplies to be used in the patient's care although hospital administration has recently issued new policies on financial management. This is known as:
   a. Role conflict
   b. Futile care
   c. Moral distress
   d. Moral courage

4. The RN takes charge of the evacuation of patients from a hospital that sustained significant storm damage and is able to get everyone to a place of safety. The nurse is demonstrating:
   a. Role conflict
   b. Futile care
   c. Moral distress
   d. Moral courage

5. The most effective way the RN can demonstrate the ethical principle of veracity is by:
   a. Not allowing protected health information to be released about the patient
   b. Helping the patient understand the nature and extent of their disease process
   c. Staying faithful to the nurse-patient relationship
   d. Providing the patient with truthful information

6. The physician expects the nurse to function in a manner that is in direct conflict with the expectations of the hospital where the nurse is employed. This is an example of:
   a. Moral distress
   b. Role conflict
   c. Nonmaleficence
   d. Values

Match the description with the correct ethical principle used in nursing.

7. ____ fair and equitable treatment for all patients

8. ____ avoiding misleading patients

9. ____ limiting the amount of information to disclose about oneself

10. ____ information that can be disclosed about a patient without his or her consent

11. ____ being loyal to commitments and accountable for responsibilities

12. ____ avoiding doing harm to the patient

13. ____ the nurse wants to do good for the patient

14. ____ the patient has the right to make their own decisions

privacy
confidentiality
veracity
fidelity
justice
nonmaleficence
beneficence
autonomy

▶ Case Study

You are a new graduate registered nurse who passed your NCLEX exam last week. You have been employed in your position as a staff nurse on a 40-bed medical floor for a month. One of the patients on the floor today is Mrs. Clark. She has been undergoing extensive testing to determine the source of persistent abdominal pain. You overhear Dr. Smith talking with Mrs. Clark's family in the hallway. You hear Dr. Smith tell the family, "Just as I thought, your mother has terminal cancer. I want to tell her as soon as possible so that she can start getting her final arrangements made." Mrs. Clark's daughter quickly responds, "Oh no, don't tell her about the cancer! We don't want her to know. Just let her think this is something you can treat." Dr. Smith reluctantly agrees to avoid telling the patient the results of the testing, at least temporarily.

1. You are very concerned about this situation. What is the ethical dilemma that exists here (*highlight in the paragraph above where the ethical dilemma exists*)?

2. Has a breach of duty occurred (*highlight in the paragraph above where the breach of duty occurred*)?

3. Which ethical principles are being violated (*select all of the responses that apply*)?
   a. Autonomy
   b. Beneficence
   c. Nonmaleficence
   d. Justice
   e. Fidelity
   f. Veracity
   g. Confidentiality
   h. Privacy

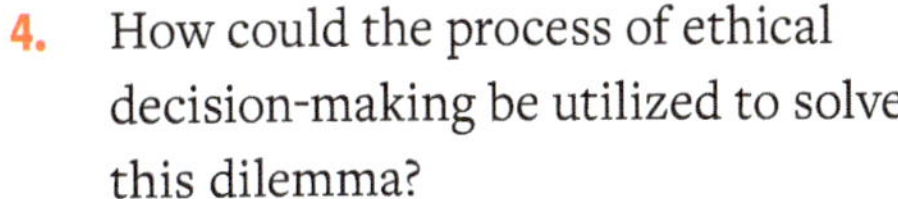

4. How could the process of ethical decision-making be utilized to solve this dilemma?

▶ Concept Map

Create a concept map that addresses Mrs. Smith's situation.

▶ Notetaker

I. Chapter introduction

   A. Ethics

   B. Values

C. Morals

II. Ethical dilemma

III. Ethical principles

A. Autonomy

B. Beneficence

C. Nonmaleficence

D. Justice

E. Fidelity

F. Veracity

G. Confidentiality

H. Privacy

IV. ANA code of ethics

V. Stages of the ethical decision-making process

A.

B.

C.

D.

E.

F.

VI. Ethical issues pertaining to death and dying

VII. Moral distress

A. Futile care

B. Moral courage

C. Situations leading to moral distress

1.

2.

3.

4.

5.

6.

References

Gallagher, A. (2010). Moral distress and moral courage in everyday nursing practice. *OJIN: Online Journal of Issues in Nursing, 16.* http://www.nursingworld.org/MainMenuCategories/ANAMarketplace/ANAPeriodicals/OJIN/TableofContents/Vol-16-2011/No2-May-2011/Articles-Previous-Topics/Moral-Distress-and-Courage-in-Everyday-Practice-.html

Huber, D. (2017). *Leadership and nursing care management* (6th ed.). Elsevier.

Pendry, P. (2007). Moral distress: Recognizing it to retain nurses. *Nursing Economics, 25,* 217–221.

Rumbold, G. (1999). *Ethics in nursing practice* (3rd ed.). Harcourt Brace and Company.

Silverman, H. J., Kheirbek, R. E., Moscou-Jackson, G., & Day, J. (2021, April). Moral distress in nurses caring for patients with COVID-19. *Nursing Ethics.*

CHAPTER

5

Legal Aspects of Nursing

CHAPTER OBJECTIVES

Upon completion of the chapter, you will be able to:

1. Discuss the different types of public law
2. Discuss the different forms of civil law
3. Describe intentional and unintentional torts
4. Discuss the importance of the Nurse Practice act
5. Describe the elements needed to prove fault on the part of a nurse charged with malpractice

KEY TERMS

administrative law
advanced directive
assault
battery
civil law
constitutional law
contract law
criminal law
defamation
durable power of attorney
encryption
false imprisonment
felony
fraud
Health Insurance Portability and Accountability Act of 1996
informed consent
invasion of privacy
libel
living will
malpractice
misdemeanor
multistate licensure compact
negligence
Nurse Practice Act
Patient Self-Determination Act
public law
slander
tort

Public Law

Public law includes constitutional law, criminal law, and administrative law (Kelly, 2010).

Constitutional law refers to a citizen's rights, privileges, and responsibilities provided through the Constitution of the United States, including those documented in the Bill of Rights. States are not allowed to pass laws that conflict with these rights because the Constitution is considered to be the highest source of American law (Zerwekh & Garneau, 2020).

Criminal law refers to actions of individuals that are intentionally directed to harm members of the public. Nurses are specifically affected by this area of law because of the mandate to protect vulnerable populations of patients. Most states require nurses to report suspected abuse of children or older adults. Failure to report such heinous acts can result in severe penalties for the health professional (Kelly, 2010).

Criminal law also affects nurses and their practice through the use of criminal background checks. Certain categories of potential employees who will work with either children or older adults, such as in day care settings and long-term care facilities, are required to have criminal background checks. Failure of a facility to implement such a requirement can result in substantial monetary loss if an employee who did not receive a background check later causes harm to a patient. It is the nurse's responsibility as the potential employee to provide accurate and truthful information to expedite the procedure. The nurse in charge of implementing background checks is responsible for ensuring the procedure is carried out thoroughly and accurately and that no prospective employee is omitted from having such a check implemented. In criminal law, the crime can be a misdemeanor or a felony. A ***misdemeanor*** is a crime of a minor nature that is punishable by a fine, a short prison term, or sometimes even both punishments. A ***felony*** is a crime of a serious nature that can be punished by a significant prison term (Kelly, 2010).

In addition, criminal law can affect the nurse and his or her practice through the stipulation that the health professional who is licensed to practice nursing cannot engage in substance abuse. Healthcare agencies that use regulated narcotic medications with their patient populations are required by both state and federal law to keep an accurate count of how these medications are used. Nurses are frequently called on to sign a record, noting the issuing of a narcotic medication to a specific patient or to serve as a witness that a partial dose of medication that was not used was destroyed. Although employing facilities can implement random drug screens of employees at any time, a nurse's employment can also be affected by use of drugs and alcohol outside of the workplace. A nurse found to be abusing drugs and/or alcohol outside of the work setting may have their employment terminated and their license either disciplined or revoked by the employing state's board of nursing (Kelly, 2010).

Finally, administrative law deals with protecting the rights of citizens. In the federal system, the Occupational Safety and Health Administration develops regulations that affect health care workers, including how hazardous substances will be stored, procedures to protect employees from infectious substances, and policies to protect employees from falling victim to workplace violence (Kelly, 2010).

Another very important part of administrative law is each state's Nurse Practice Act. Each state's Nurse Practice Act gives that state's board of nursing the authority to define:

- How nursing will be practiced in that locale
- Educational preparation required to practice as either a licensed practical/vocational nurse or registered nurse in that state
- How professional nurses will be disciplined if they do not adhere to the rules governing nursing practice

In addition, each state's board of nursing determines if that state will agree to recognize nursing licenses from other states, such as occurs through the multistate licensure compact. The multistate licensure compact allows an agreement to be developed between specific states to enable nurses licensed in one state to practice in another state without being required to apply for a new license. However, as of 2011 only 24 states have opted to participate in the multistate licensure compact, thus indicating the level of concern centered on this area of administrative law (Huynh & Haddad, 2021).

Civil Law

In addition to public law, the nurse can be affected by civil law. ***Civil law*** refers to how individuals relate to each other in daily life and consists of both contract law and tort law. **Contract law** regulates certain types of transactions between individuals and businesses and between businesses. For an agreement to be recognized as a legal contract, it must contain the following points:

- Must be agreed on by two or more legally competent individuals or parties and must state what each party must or must not do
- Mutual understanding of the stipulations imposed on each party involved in the contract
- Some type of payment given in exchange for the actions that were taken or not taken as part of implementing the contract

The nurse can be affected by contract as an employee. The nurse who is employed agrees to adhere to the facility's policies and procedures, fulfills the duties of the employer that have already been agreed on by both parties, and respects the rights and responsibilities of the other employees working in the facility. In addition, the employer agrees to pay the nurse a specific amount for services rendered, give the nurse adequate assistance in providing care, provide the supplies and equipment needed to fulfill required responsibilities, and provide reasonable treatment and behavior from the other health care providers who will be interacting with the nurse in the work environment (Kelly, 2010).

Another form of civil law is tort law. A **tort** is a negligent or intentional wrong not connected with a contract that injures a person and for which the injured party may opt to sue the responsible person for damages. Torts commonly include denying a person his or her legal rights, failing to comply with public duties, and failing to perform a duty owed to a person that results in harm occurring to another person. Torts can be intentional or unintentional. Examples of intentional torts are **assault** and **battery**. Assault consists of threatening to touch another person, such as a patient, in a manner that is offensive to that person and without their permission. Battery consists of actually carrying out the threat and proceeding to touch the person without having their permission. In addition, fraud, defamation, false imprisonment, and invasion of privacy could be considered to be intentional torts. ***Fraud*** is false representation of a fact because you are aware that it will be acted upon by someone else. An example of this would be falsifying your academic credentials on your resume to deceive a potential employer. In comparison, ***defamation*** is a disregard for the truth that can damage another person's reputation. Defamation can be further subdivided into libel and slander. ***Libel*** is defamation that occurs through printing, writing, or use of pictures. ***Slander*** is defamation that is spoken. In addition, ***false imprisonment*** is restraining a person against his wishes. An example of this could be preventing a competent person from leaving the hospital. ***Invasion of privacy*** occurs when a nurse intrudes on a patient's private affairs. An example of this would be photographing a patient's wound without getting permission.

Examples of unintentional torts are malpractice or negligence. Malpractice consists of a professional's wrongful conduct in carrying out their duties as a professional, leading to harm ensuing to another person entrusted to their care. Negligence, in comparison, consists of failing to provide the care that a reasonable professional would provide in a similar situation. If a nurse is charged with malpractice or negligence, damages can only be recovered if fault on the part of the nurse can be proven. For fault to be proven, the following areas must be shown (Kelly, 2010):

- Duty: This is the obligation of the nurse to exercise the kind of care that a reasonable prudent nurse would use.
- Breach of duty: This is the failure to meet the standard of care.
- Causation: There is a failure to meet the standard of care that results in harm to the patient.
- Damages: The client experiences actual harm or injury.

Advanced Directives

The registered nurse (RN) must have an understanding of how the concept of advanced directives affects the patient. An advanced directive is a set of instructions that give a person's wishes related to their health care if they were unable to make and verbalize a decision. Educating patients about advance directives is required by the Patient Self-Determination Act. This legislation also requires that patients be given the opportunity to complete an advance directive if so desired (Wilkinson & Treas, 2019).

There are two types of advance directives the RN may be required to discuss with a patient: the living will and the durable power of attorney. The living will is a document prepared by a competent person that gives instructions about the medical care that should be provided for that person if they become unable to make and verbalize decisions. Also specified are the types of health care a person would not want at the end of their life, such as specifying that they do not want to receive tube feedings. In comparison, the durable power of attorney exists when a competent person names another person to make decisions about their health care when unable to do so. The document frequently gives specific instructions about feeding tubes, cardiopulmonary resuscitation, and being placed on ventilators. Such a document must be witnessed by two people (Wilkinson & Treas, 2019).

Informed Consent

Informed consent is the legal right of the patient to receive accurate and adequate information that pertains to a medical condition or treatment. The law assumes that an adult patient will have the capacity to make an informed decision about a choice of treatment. If a court deems a patient to be incapable of making an informed decision, it may appoint a guardian to make decisions on the patient's behalf. A parent or legal guardian will provide the informed consent for minor children. The exception to this is a minor who is married or who has gone to court to become emancipated. The responsibility for providing the patient with the information needed to give informed consent rests with the physician. The nurse is responsible for witnessing the patient's signature on the form once the nurse can verify that the patient understands the information provided by the physician (Wilkinson & Treas, 2019).

Issues Involving Confidentiality

All patient information must be kept private and confidential. The Health Insurance Portability and Accountability Act of 1996 (HIPAA) first brought privacy issues involving medical information to the public's attention in its year of adoption. The legislation includes a system for ensuring privacy regarding health information that could potentially be used to identify a specific patient. Information used to provide treatment, payment, or any type of health care operation does not require a patient's specific consent for it to be used. This means a patient can be billed for a surgical procedure without having to give consent for "surgical procedure" to be typed onto the remittance slip. However, disclosure of any type of medical information must be of the bare minimum amount, only what is absolutely necessary. The patient must be notified of how the information will be used (Zerwekh & Garneau, 2020).

Additional requirements were added to HIPAA in 2005. These stipulated that to ensure that protected patient information is disclosed only on a need-to-know basis, each institution must conduct its own risk assessment and develop data security policies and technologies in response to the assessment. The facility may opt to have information coded or encrypted when it is sent over the Internet to ensure it is not accessed by someone who does not have a right to view it (Zerwekh & Garneau, 2020).

To ensure continuity of care for patients continues despite the HIPAA requirements, some states have enacted legislation to protect communication that occurs between health care providers and patients. This means that information can be communicated freely between physicians and patients without fear of it falling into the wrong person's access. Usually such a privilege is extended to nurses as well as physicians. Ultimately, however, it is the RN's responsibility to maintain confidentiality any time they have access to patient information. Such sensitive information should not be discussed with coworkers in the elevator where the public could overhear it or at home with the nurse's family members. Maintaining such a practice cannot only help avoid a lawsuit for the RN but can also allow the nurse to serve as a mentor and role model for new graduate nurses (Zerwekh & Garneau, 2020).

▶ Summary of Key Points in Chapter

Although this chapter discussed legal aspects of nursing, a wide variety of topics was presented. This included a discussion of the various types of public law (constitutional law, criminal law, and administrative law) and civil law (contract law and tort law). Under public law, the importance of administrative law's creation of state boards of nursing was emphasized. The significance of the types of advance directives as well as HIPAA to the RN was reviewed.

▶ Conclusion

This chapter has shown multiple legal issues at work in the modern health care environment, and most of them will, at some point, influence the RN and the care that is delivered to patients and their support systems. It is the responsibility of the RN who is transitioning into the process of becoming a nurse leader to stay up-to-the-minute with all available information on new developments in the legal arena that could affect not only the nurse's practice but the facility where that practice occurs.

Legal issues can be further complicated by the nurse's failure to develop cultural competence. The thoughtless use of stereotyping rather than the development of cultural understanding and empathy for vulnerable populations can prove to be a serious barrier to appropriate health care delivery. The development of cultural competence and its importance for the emerging nurse leader will be discussed in the subsequent chapter.

▶ Critical Thinking Questions

1. Compare and contrast the major characteristics of constitutional, criminal, and administrative law.

2. Think about your own work environment and identify a situation that involved:

   a. Constitutional law

   b. Criminal law

c. Administrative law

d. How was each situation resolved?

e. Do you believe any individual's rights were violated?

f. At any point were patients endangered?

3. Compare and contrast the major points of contract law and tort law.

4. Describe how the RN can expect to be affected by:

a. Constitutional law

b. Criminal law

c. Administrative law

d. Contract law

e. Tort law

5. Compare and contrast the major points of negligence and malpractice.

6. How can the RN expect to be affected by their state's Nurse Practice Act?

7. How would you explain the concepts of the living will and durable power of attorney to:

    a. A physician who is undergoing surgery?

    b. A nurse who is undergoing surgery?

    c. A mechanic with an eighth-grade education who is undergoing surgery?

    d. An immigrant who can speak and understand simple English but cannot read or write English?

▶ Scenarios

1. You are the nursing supervisor for a large hospital. While making rounds in the hospital one evening, you identify a nurse who appears to be intoxicated.

    a. What is the best action for you to implement at this time?

    b. What is the best action for you to implement in 24 hours?

2. You are in charge of supervising the background check procedure for your hospital. You are notified that a prospective employee who is also a nurse has refused to submit to a background check.

   a. What is your best action at this time?

   b. The nurse in the scenario above agrees to submit to the background check but fails it.

   c. What is your best course of action now?

3. You are the director of nursing for a large hospital. You are notified that one of your employees, a nurse, failed a random urine drug test.

   a. What is your best course of action now?

   b. What is your long-term plan for this employee?

4. You are the director of nursing for a large metropolitan hospital. You are informed that one of the nurses in the facility left the facility after being pulled to another floor to work for the day and accepting a patient assignment on that floor.

    a. What are the legal implications of this nurse's decision?

    b. What should be your highest priority action after being informed of the situation?

5. You are the director of nursing of a large metropolitan hospital. You are informed that a patient has complained to the state board of nursing that a nurse employed with your facility struck him while providing care.

    a. What are the legal implications of this information?

b. What should be your highest priority action as director of nursing?

6. You are informed that an investigator from the state board of nursing has attempted to contact you as the facility director of nursing to get information about the nurse who has had a complaint brought against her license.

   a. What should be your highest-priority action?

   b. If the board of nursing judges there is sufficient cause to pursue the investigation with the nurse, how do you anticipate the process will proceed?

7. You are mentoring a new graduate nurse who expresses concern about giving report to the oncoming shift. He asks you, "Legally, are we allowed to do this? Isn't this a HIPAA violation?"

   a. What should be your response?

   b. How can you explain to him the major points of the HIPAA law?

▸ NCLEX-Style Review Questions

1. An RN is found to be guilty of discriminating against a patient based on that patient's religion. Under the state Nurse Practice Act, the nurse is likely to have discipline brought against their license based on:
   a. Criminal conviction
   b. Unprofessional conduct
   c. Unethical/unprofessional practice
   d. Unsafe practice

2. An RN is found to be guilty of embezzling funds. Under the state Nurse Practice Act, the nurse is likely to have discipline brought against their license based on:
   a. Criminal conviction
   b. Unprofessional conduct
   c. Unethical/unprofessional practice
   d. Unsafe practice

3. An RN is found to be guilty of negligence in their nursing practice. Under the state Nurse Practice Act, the nurse is likely to have discipline brought against their license based on:
   a. Criminal conviction
   b. Unprofessional conduct
   c. Unethical/unprofessional practice
   d. Unsafe practice

4. An RN is found to be guilty of obtaining a nursing license using a false name. Under the state Nurse Practice Act, the nurse is likely to have discipline brought against their license based on:
   a. Criminal conviction
   b. Unprofessional conduct
   c. Unethical/unprofessional practice
   d. Unsafe practice

5. The RN notes that his patient's chart now includes a document that names another person who can make decisions about the patient's health care if she is unable to do so. The RN recognizes this document as a(n):
   a. Living will
   b. Durable power of attorney
   c. Advanced directive
   d. Patient self-determination

6. The RN finds that his patient is asking for information on how to provide some basic instructions on his wishes for health care if he is unable to verbalize what he wants done for himself. The RN recognizes the patient needs to complete a(n):
   a. Living will
   b. Durable power of attorney
   c. Advanced directive
   d. Patient self-determination

7. The RN is caring for a patient who arrived at the hospital with a document naming another person to make decisions about her health care if she is unable to do so. The document also provides information describing the circumstances under which the person would want a feeding tube as well as ventilator placement. The RN recognizes that this is a(n):
   a. Living will
   b. Durable power of attorney
   c. Advanced directive
   d. Patient self-determination

▶ Case Study

You are a new graduate nurse working on a large medical-surgical floor. One of your colleagues, Sue, is caring for Mrs. Smith, an 84-year-old female patient who is being treated for end-stage breast cancer. Sue comes to the nurse's station and sits next to you as she begins to work on shift documentation. She tells you, "I finally got Mrs. Smith to take her medication for the shift. I'm so glad that's over." You respond, "That's great! I know that she really hates the side effects of that medication. How did you convince her to take it?"

Sue tells you, "It was easy! I told her that the doctor would send her to a nursing home if she didn't take it."

Later, as you pass by Mrs. Smith's room, you hear her crying.

1. The type of law involved in this scenario is ______________: *(select all that apply)*
   a. Public law
   b. Civil law
   c. Contract law
   d. Constitutional law
   e. Criminal law
   f. Administrative law

2. Was there a breach of duty on Sue's part? *(highlight in the paragraph above where the breach of duty took place)*

3. What could you do to assist the patient? (*select all that apply*)
   a. Tell the patient that Sue was correct about her transfer to a nursing home
   b. Talk with the physician about ways to lessen the medication side effects
   c. Comfort the patient and listen to her concerns
   d. Question the patient about the side effects of the medication
   e. Talk with the patient about potentially refusing further chemotherapeutic agents
   f. Talk with the patient's family about transferring her to a nursing home
4. What should you say to your colleague regarding this situation?

▶ Concept Map

Create a concept map that is reflective of Mrs. Smith's situation.

Note Taker

I. Public law

II. Criminal law

A. Misdemeanor

B. Felony

III. Administrative law

IV. Civil law

A. Intentional torts

1. Assault

2. Battery

3. Fraud

4. Defamation

5. Libel

6. Slander

7. False imprisonment

8. Invasion of privacy

B. Unintentional torts

1. Malpractice

2. Negligence

3. Duty

4. Breach of duty

5. Causation

6. Damages

V. Advanced directives

A. Patient Self-Determination Act

B. Living will

C. Durable power of attorney

VI. Informed consent

VII. Health Insurance Portability and Affordability Act of 1996

References

Huynh, A. P., & Haddad, L. M. *Nursing Practice Act* [updated 2021 Jul 22]. In: StatPearls [Internet]. Treasure Island (FL): StatPearls Publishing; 2021 Jan-. https://www.ncbi.nlm.nih.gov/books/NBK559012

Kelly, P., & Tazbir, J. (2021). *Essentials of nursing leadership and management* (4th ed.). Delmar.

Wilkinson, J., & Treas, L. (2019). *Fundamentals of nursing* (4th ed.). F. A. Davis.

Zerwekh, J., & Garneau, A. (2020). *Nursing today: Transitions and trends* (10th ed.). Elsevier.

CHAPTER

6

Cultural Aspects of Nursing

KEY TERMS

acculturation
assimilation
biomedical view
cultural humility
culture
culture shock
diversity
health equity
Healthy People 2030
holistic view
inclusion
magico-religious view
socialization
vulnerable populations

CHAPTER OBJECTIVES

Upon completion of the chapter, you will be able to:

1. Discuss the various factors that make up an individual's culture
2. Describe the various ways a registered nurse can increase their cultural humility
3. Describe beliefs of various cultural or ethnic groups that could affect delivery of nursing care
4. Discuss the concepts unique to the model of cultural humility in health care delivery
5. Describe the process of conducting a cultural assessment on a patient

Introduction

The registered nurse (RN) transitioning into the health care community as a nurse leader must be able to function in not only the local hospital but also what is increasingly known as the "global society." Americans in particular are multicultural to such an extent that the RN must develop cultural humility to provide adequate nursing care. The nurse who fails to see the importance of being sensitive to a patient's primary language, ethnicity, cultural beliefs, gender identification, and racial makeup will inevitably provide substandard care because a rapport cannot be built between the nurse and the patient. Nurses must be able to have an understanding of health care disparities and how they can be reduced to provide care to vulnerable populations. Increasingly, the RN in the modern health care system must recognize the importance of encouraging diversity in the nursing workforce that mirrors the diversity seen in the global society. Health equity must be a priority of all health care workers to ensure that all individuals have equal access to the information needed to make informed choices about their health care. Finally, it is essential that America's health care workforce become as diverse as possible. Health care as a workforce should be as inclusive as possible to ensure that it represents our country's makeup regarding race/ethnicity, gender, sexual orientation, immigration status, physical disability status, and socioeconomic level so that patients receive the highest possible quality in the health care provided and are assured that their needs are met (Stanford, 2020).

Cultural Humility

Cultural humility may be thought of as the process of being aware of how an individual's culture can impact health behaviors and then using this awareness to develop sensitivity in treating patients. Cultural humility begins with self-reflection. As the nurse begins the process of developing cultural humility, the patient's culture must be carefully considered (Prasad et al., 2016). Cultural humility can also be thought of as the ability to remain open to another person's identity, recognizing that the person's cultural background, beliefs, values, and traditions will impact how the individual makes decisions about care being received. In addition, cultural humility involves recognition of power imbalances. For example, the patient may believe that health care recommendations from a medical practitioner must be accepted without question even though this is not the case. Cultural humility also considers institutional accountability as part of the process of ensuring that the most appropriate care options are available to all patients. Hospitals and other health care facilities can take responsibility for differences in care and can work to change inequitable policies (Caba & Colon, n.d.).

How can cultural humility affect patients and their treatment options?

- A significant health issue can change the patient's household structure so that adult children may need to care for an aging parent or one partner may need to care for another, for example. Changes in the household may conflict with traditions in the client's community.
- Certain belief systems may connect past actions to a significant diagnosis. This can lead the patient to be reluctant to share a diagnosis with members of the individual's support network.
- Some cultural groups have beliefs that would lead them to decline treatment options such as blood transfusions or reconstructive surgery. Although this may be difficult for medical personnel to understand, the patient must be acknowledged as making the ultimate decision regarding such treatment options.
- Some communities do not view discussing end-of-life issues while the patient is still alive as being appropriate. This may lead patients to be reluctant to discuss estate planning or funeral arrangements even though they recognize the necessity of this.
- The individual's culture usually has defined rituals centered around grief and mourning. Grief may be expressed privately rather than publicly. The person may seem to be more concerned about family dynamics and a decrease in income than about the impending loss of the patient (Caba & Colon, n.d.).

How can nurses encourage themselves to develop cultural humility? Caba & Colon (n.d.) have developed the following series of questions, which nurses can ask themselves to provoke the development of cultural humility:

- What kind of support does the patient need from the nurse?

- What kind of support does the patient need from other members of the health care community?
- How can the nurse draw the patient into the conversation about the individual's care?
- What assumptions is the nurse making? How can the nurse learn more about situations involving the patient that are not immediately obvious?
- If the nurse has difficulty understanding the patient's viewpoint, which questions can the nurse ask to understand more?
- How can the nurse validate the choices that the patient is making?

Overview of Culture

An individual's culture is the interwoven pattern of behavior composed of elements such as:

- Language
- Thoughts
- Mode of communication
- Actions
- Customs
- Belief system
- Values
- Institutions unique to racial and ethnic makeup
- Religious and social groups

In addition, several factors characterize culture as a concept (Wilkinson & Treas, 2019):

- Culture is learned: The individual learns how to view their life and role in it through the other members of the culture. Frequently, the culture's older members provide instruction to the younger members.
- Culture is taught: The values and beliefs usually are passed down from one generation to the next, with some younger members accepting the traditional practices and others choosing not to see the value of such teaching.
- Culture is shared by its members: As social interaction occurs with all members of the culture, the concepts that are unique to the culture are passed back and forth.
- Culture is constantly changing: Cultural beliefs and practices change over time; change can occur in response to the culture's environment. This could occur if a culture loses its traditional homeland because of war in the home country.
- Culture is complex: Many cultural concepts occur at an unconscious level and may be difficult for members of the culture to verbalize.
- Culture is diverse: Variety exists among members of a particular cultural group.
- Culture is multilevel: Culture consists of both a material level composed of art, literature, costumes, and artifacts and a nonmaterial level composed of traditions, language, beliefs, and practices.
- Culture is sharing beliefs and practices: For a practice or belief to be considered cultural in nature, it must be shared by the majority of the members of a culture.

- Culture is influential: The culture should be capable of influencing all aspects of members' lives.
- Culture is identifying: Cultural beliefs can provide a sense of belonging for the members even if the culture involved is a subculture; however, if the beliefs of the subculture conflict with the beliefs of the primary culture, the subculture can prove to be a detrimental influence on the members.

These factors that form an individual's culture are significant to such an extent that they affect the way in which the person thinks, processes a problem to solve it, and views the world and the way it is structured. Culture is a valuable part of a society because of its ability to communicate past experiences of the group and thus ensure traditions are passed from one generation to the next. This significance can be shown by the culture shock that develops when a person emigrates from one culture to another and finds their belief system and values are not highly esteemed by the new culture (Kelly & Tazbir, 2013).

In a society, in addition to the major cultural group to which all individuals belong, we all also belong to multiple smaller subcultures, each with its own belief system and values and expectations for its members. Subcultures you may belong to as a RN may include:

- Professional affiliations
- Age group
- Socioeconomic level
- Political affiliation

A person admitted into the modern health care system may also experience culture shock, as they become part of a culture and experience new words, frightening sights, strange odors, and a never-ending stream of strangers entering their personal space. Such culture shock increases greatly when the patient also does not speak English as his or her primary language (Kelly & Tazbir, 2013).

Functioning as a Culture

How does a culture actually function in modern society? We must recognize initially that, as noted in the previous discussion regarding subcultures, almost no one belongs to only one cultural group. Just as most areas of the United States are multicultural because they are populated by people from a wide variety of cultural groups, hospitals and other health care environments are multicultural. They are filled with people from various subcultures, including nurses, physicians, nursing assistants, respiratory therapists, nursing students, and patients' family members, to name only a few. All these individuals are from various ethnic groups, races, and religious groups and serve a variety of roles in society. As these groups gain new members, those individuals must be socialized into the group by learning how to function as a member of this cultural group. The nursing student learns how to conduct themselves in the clinical setting, in the classroom, and with other students (Wilkinson & Treas, 2019).

This process can be more difficult for the person who joins a new cultural group as an immigrant from another country. The immigrant must adopt the characteristics of the new culture through acculturation, thus assuming aspects of both cultures. This ensures survival in the new culture associated with the new country. Some experts have estimated that an immigrant group may require three generations to become acculturated.

Some immigrant groups take the process one step further to assimilation, in which these individuals choose to learn about and assume the values, beliefs, and behaviors of the primary culture of the nation. You could be spoken of as assimilated into French culture, for example, if you moved to France, learned to speak French, began working in the French health care system, became close friends with several French citizens, and learned the French style of cooking (Wilkinson & Treas, 2019).

Vulnerable Populations

Vulnerable populations are groups of individuals who are likely to develop health problems and experience poor outcomes in response to nursing interventions and medical treatment as a result of diminished access to medical care, various types of stressors, and engaging in types of high-risk behavior. Such groups can include the following:

- Homeless individuals
- Individuals living below the poverty line
- People experiencing mental illness
- People with various types of physical disabilities and challenges
- Children
- Older adults

Some ethnic and racial minorities are considered to be vulnerable populations because of the known prevalence of various disease processes among them. For example, African Americans are known to have a high rate of hypertension, osteoporosis is prevalent among small-framed White women, and Native Americans and Alaska Natives are known to be vulnerable to develop diabetes (Wilkinson & Treas, 2019).

Healthy People 2030

Healthy People 2030 was developed by the U.S. Department of Health and Human Services (DHHS; 2022) in an attempt to address the gaps in care for vulnerable populations and ultimately to decrease the existing health disparities in America. The project consists of a set of goals and objectives with a 10-year target designed to guide health promotion and disease prevention on a national scale. The basic premise of the initiative is that the combination of goal setting and evidence-based benchmarks can be used to motivate individuals and focus actions designed to improve their health. Healthy People 2030 and its previous versions has been used by the federal government, state governments, and individual communities to measure the progress in resolving health issues in certain vulnerable populations (DHHS, 2022).

As a public health initiative, Healthy People 2030 identified a mission, as follows (DHHS, 2022):

- Identify priorities for improving individuals' health throughout the United States.

- Increase public awareness of what determines health, disease, and disabling conditions, as well as opportunities to resolve disease processes.
- Develop measurable goals and objectives that are useful at the national, state, and community levels.
- Involve multiple personnel to act to strengthen policies and improve evidence-based practices.
- Identify research, evaluation, and data collection priorities.

In addition, the primary goals of Healthy People 2030 are identified as follows:

- Attain lives of greater longevity and higher quality that have no evidence of preventable disease, disability, injury, or premature death.
- Achieve equity in health, eliminate evidence of health disparities, and improve the health status of all vulnerable populations.
- Create both social and physical environments that promote an overall increased level of health for all individuals involved.
- Promote the increased quality of life, healthy development, and health-promoting behaviors across all stages of the life span.

The mission and goals of Healthy People 2030 affect the RN nurse leader who is providing care in today's health care community. The non-Hispanic White population is projected to shrink over the coming decades, from 199 million in 2020 to 179 million people in 2060. The population of people who are two or more races is projected to be the fastest-growing racial or ethnic group over the next several decades, followed by Asians and Hispanics. The nation's foreign-born population is projected to rise from 44 million people in 2016 to 69 million in 2060, growing from about 14% to 17% of the population (Vespa et al, 2020). These figures suggest that modern nurses must be prepared to care for individuals who may reap the benefits of modern medicine in terms of longevity and treatability of conditions but also may speak English as a second language.

Need for Health Equity

The increasing need for health equity can be clearly illustrated by reviewing the leading causes of death for Caucasian Americans and African Americans. The Centers for Disease Control and Prevention (CDC; 2022) noted that for all ages of non-Hispanic Caucasian males, the top five causes of death in 2018 were heart disease, cancer, unintentional injuries, chronic lower respiratory disease, and stroke. In comparison, the CDC noted that the top five causes of death for African American males of all ages consisted of heart disease, cancer, Alzheimer's disease, stroke, and homicide.

Some foreign-born individuals may receive fewer routine immunizations, use preventive healthcare less frequently, develop some infectious diseases such as tuberculosis at a significantly higher rate, and delay seeking treatment for some infectious disease processes. The health status of immigrants is further challenged by the pressures of adjusting to a new dominant culture; finding employment, particularly when the individual is undocumented; and learning to communicate in a new language (Truman et al., 2009).

Other particularly vulnerable populations are immigrants and refugees. These groups are believed to be particularly vulnerable to the development of pandemic influenza. The number of foreign-born individuals living in the United States is projected to increase from 12% in 2005 to 15% in 2015. In 2009, this number amounted to approximately 38 million individuals (Morello & Keating, 2009). When compared with individuals born in the United States, foreign-born individuals are more likely to live in poverty, less likely to have a high school diploma, and less likely to have health care coverage.

Undocumented individuals are most likely to experience barriers to access to health care, because these people tend to avoid contact with public officials due to fear of deportation. Foreign-born individuals are known to have a higher prevalence of diabetes, infections, and occupational injuries than American-born residents of the same race and ethnic origin (Truman et al., 2009).

The implications for recognizing that such health problems exist in vulnerable populations are great. There are several strategies to resolve such disparities, such as those that follow (Baldwin, 2003):

- Develop prevention programs in the community that involve working with and being connected to a facility; this ensures patients can readily have lab work drawn or nutritional counseling implemented.
- Use the strategies for prevention that have already been discussed; regardless of your role in the overall health care continuum, the primary prevention strategies can be practiced by everyone.
- Promote wellness and a healthy lifestyle; be mindful that the health care professional must have completed a full assessment of the cultural beliefs and practices of the vulnerable population in question before implementing wellness prevention, as some Western strategies might prove offensive to other cultures.
- Be mindful of the personal choices of individuals and the existing social environment, particularly interactions with family, acquaintances, and the community; it may prove helpful to involve entire families or even communities in educational sessions.
- Make the effort to provide patients with complete information without seeming to rush the interaction; members of vulnerable populations frequently note that health care professionals seem rushed in their interaction with patients, and members of other cultures often find this offensive.

Once the nurse has made the effort to understand the cultural beliefs of the patient, the process of communication can begin. The following cultural-related factors will affect communication with the patient (D'Amico & Barbarito, 2015):

- Dominant spoken and written language: According to census data released in 2007, 20% of the American population spoke a language other than English (Ohlemacher, 2007). Furthermore, even among English-speaking individuals, there are differences in word use and pronunciation, and various tones of voice can be considered more significant than others.
- Methods of nonverbal communication: These include gestures, facial expressions, and various types of mannerisms. Emotions can be communicated nonverbally through the

use of silence, touch, eye contact or failure to make eye contact, moving away from others during the process of communication, and posture of the speaker or listener. It is important to recognize which cultures value silence as demonstrating respect for another individual and which ones use silence to indicate interest in the speaker's words. Also, some cultures do not allow casual touch and also have strict requirements regarding personal space. Some have specific rules regarding what type of touch is considered to be appropriate for members of the opposite gender.

- Time orientation: A culture may have unique views of the past, present, and future. Whereas European Americans view time in terms of punctuality and scheduling, other cultures are not as future-oriented. For example, some Native Americans consider time primarily in terms of the past. Time is important to them because of the traditional practices that have been passed down through generations from their ancestors. In comparison, some Hispanic cultures do not view time as significant.
- Family roles and relationships: The specified roles and relationships in the patient's family relate to how decision-making is valued and implemented, the culture's view of age, and specific views of each gender. Some cultures are more likely to follow a patriarchal pattern of decision-making, whereas others tend to consult the matriarchal member of the family for assistance with decision-making.
- Nutritional intake: The patient's daily diet may be culturally determined. Specific foods may be eaten at specific times or as part of cultural ritualistic practices. The RN should familiarize themselves with as many of these as possible because they can significantly affect the patient's treatment and recovery process:
  - Americans typically have coffee in the morning with breakfast.
  - Muslims fast from dawn to sunset during the month of Ramadan as part of their religious practice.
  - Roman Catholics observe Lent by eating one full meal and two small meals on Ash Wednesday and Good Friday and avoid eating meat on Ash Wednesday and Fridays until Easter as part of their religious practice.
  - Muslims avoid eating pork.
  - Jews may practice kosher dietary laws.
  - Mexican, Iranian, Chinese, and Vietnamese cultures all view achieving the balance between hot and cold foods as both a method of preventing illness and a method of treating illness.
- Types of health beliefs and health practices: Health beliefs typically fall into one of three types: magico-religious, biomedical, or holistic. The magico-religious view holds that health and illness are the result of supernatural intervention. The biomedical view proposes that illness is caused by germs, viruses, or some type of breakdown in the basic functioning of the body. The holistic view proposes that illness results from a person's life failing to be in harmony with nature.

Summary of Key Points in Chapter

The chapter discussed various aspects of assessing and caring for a patient of another culture. The factors that make up the concept of culture were reviewed as well as the need for cultural humility from the RN. In addition, ways for the nurse to increase cultural humility in providing care to the patient were discussed.

Finally, the health disparities present in various vulnerable populations of patients were described, specifically the cultural or ethnic minorities of:

- The African American population
- The Hispanic population
- The immigrant/refugee population

Conclusion

Regardless of the role implemented in the modern health care facility or simply in the current health care continuum, today's RN has surely noted that they are serving the current health care customer in a global society. The RN in a busy metropolitan hospital is just as likely to be working with a patient from Nigeria as one from the local community. Without such knowledge, the professional will lack the ability to quickly detect health problems in a patient's societal group and may inadvertently allow a patient to do without much-needed health care.

A huge part of working with patients from other cultures is establishing the nurse-patient relationship, which is forged on the trust that the patient has in the abilities of the nurse. This trust will develop as the nurse cares for the patient consistently and accurately. Much of this trust will grow as the patient observes the nurse providing care utilizing sophisticated techniques such as those implemented through informatics. Informatics and its relationship to the modern RN will be discussed in the subsequent chapter.

Critical Thinking Questions

1. List as many things as you can that make up your own individual culture.

2. Describe an incident when you experienced culture shock and your reaction to it.

3. Try to list all the subcultures to which you belong.

4. Look at the list of the subcultures you developed in the previous question. How has being part of each subculture affected your beliefs and values?

5. Consider your current or former work environment or a clinical situation.
   a. Can you recall a time when you observed a patient experiencing culture shock?
   b. What was the outcome of this experience?

6. Consider the most effective way to resolve the following situations: Your patient is complaining he is unable to obtain the type of dietary intake that meets the requirements of his culture while he is hospitalized. What can you do to resolve this so that the patient receives the food that is culturally correct?

   a. What can you do to resolve this so that the dietary staff understands what is culturally appropriate for the patient's dietary intake?

   b. What can you do to resolve this so that the patient's family is involved in planning the patient's dietary intake?

   c. What can you do to resolve this so that the hospital does not go to an excessive amount of expense because of the patient's cultural dietary requirements?

7. The hospital where you work or have your clinical rotation cannot afford to either hire a trained interpreter to work with its large population of Korean-speaking patients or send an employee for the required training needed. You are the nurse manager of the medical floor where many of the Korean-speaking patients usually are admitted.

    a. What can you do to communicate with these patients more effectively?

    b. You find that the number of Korean-speaking patients admitted to your floor is increasing. What resources can you find in your community that would help you communicate more effectively with these patients and also help you understand the culture?

    c. The one nurse in the facility who speaks fluent Spanish where you are employed or have your clinical rotation is out on medical leave. A tour bus with 20 Spanish-speaking tourists has been involved in an accident, and 12 passengers have been brought to your hospital's emergency department. What can you do to most effectively communicate with patients in this situation?

    d. How can you most effectively perform triage in the emergency department with this large group of Spanish-speaking patients?

▶ Scenarios

1. You are caring for a 21-year-old Hispanic woman admitted to the medical floor where you have your clinical rotation after gashing her leg badly in a car accident. At her bedside is her 30-year-old husband who is assuming the role of interpreter. The patient understands most English that is spoken to her but can speak very little. She has been able to communicate with you so far that she is in a great deal of pain and is concerned about her three children, who are ages 4, 3, and 6 months. What can the nurse do to communicate effectively with the patient and his family?

2. You are caring for a patient who is a 48-year-old Pacific Islander. He is a newly diagnosed diabetic, is 25 pounds overweight, and is married and has two children, ages 14 and 10. He seems very depressed even though the physician believes the diabetes is easily treatable with diet and exercise. What can the nurse do to communicate effectively with the patient and his family?

3. You are working with a 58-year-old female Chinese patient who is experiencing episodes of severe abdominal pain. She arrives at the health clinical accompanied by her husband, her married daughter, and her grandchildren. The entire family is very concerned and anxious about her situation. What can you do to communicate effectively with this patient and her family?

4. A 72-year-old Japanese patient is brought to the emergency department after sustaining a massive heart attack. When talking with the family, you discover the patient has been experiencing pain for at least the past two weeks and self-medicating with acupuncture treatments. What should you do to communicate effectively with this patient and his family?

5. A 21-year-old Hindu woman is brought into the emergency department after attempting suicide. She is accompanied by her mother who acknowledges that the girl has been experiencing symptoms of depression since being notified that a traditional marriage was being arranged for her by her father. What should you do to communicate effectively with this patient and her family?

6. You are caring for a 48-year-old Hispanic woman who is refusing to receive treatment for ovarian cancer. She tells you the cancer is God's judgment on her for separating from her husband two years ago. What should you do to communicate effectively with this patient and her family?

7. You need to teach a Native American patient how to perform a dressing change on his leg wound. The dressing procedure will need to change over the next two weeks as the wound progressively heals. What is the best way to teach this patient how to perform the dressing change and care for his leg wound?

8. You are working with a Japanese patient who is recovering from a severe burn. He is refusing opioid pain medication even when he clearly is in severe discomfort. What should you do to communicate effectively with this patient and his family?

9. You are working with an Orthodox Jewish client who observes kosher dietary practices. Which factors do you believe will affect your communication with this patient?

10. You are working with a Muslim patient. Which factors do you believe will affect your communication with this patient?

11. You are working with a Native American patient. Which factors do you believe will affect your communication with this patient?

12. You are working with a Chinese patient who is also blind. Which factors do you believe will affect your communication with this patient?

▶ NCLEX-Style Review Questions

Match the cultural/spiritual belief with the appropriate cultural/ethnic group. More than one group can be selected if appropriate.

1. ____ The oldest male may serve as the decision-maker for the family.
2. ____ The patient will tend to think only in the present.
3. ____ The disease is the result of an imbalance in the patient's "hot" and "cold."
4. ____ A trusting relationship must be established with the health care provider before the patient will accept their assistance.
5. ____ The patient may try various home remedies before seeking out Western medicine.
6. ____ Illness is divine intervention in response to sinful behavior.
7. ____ Older family members are consulted about decisions involved in health and illness.

8. ____ The patient may avoid acknowledging family members' evidence of mental illness or intellectual disability out of fear that it will affect the chance of their other family members' ability to marry.

9. ____ The patient will have difficulty with instructions regarding something to do in the future.

10. ____ Illness can be the result of inadequate diet or lack of sleep.

11. ____ Illness can be prevented through the use of nutrition, herbs, rest, cleanliness, and laxative use.

12. ____ The patient is in a healthy state when in harmony with nature.

13. ____ Illness can be prevented through the use of both copper and silver bracelets.

14. ____ Illness occurs when there is a balance between the patient and nature or the supernatural.

15. ____ Time is not significant.

16. ____ Hot and cold foods can be used as a method of preventing and treating illness.

17. ____ A medicine man or woman may be consulted before health care providers are utilized.

18. ____ Time is viewed as being primarily in the past.

19. ____ A primary family member may be consulted when significant health-related decisions must be made.

20. ____ Herbalists and spiritual healers are used along with physicians.

a. African American
b. Chinese
c. Japanese
d. Hindu/Muslim
e. Vietnamese
f. Hispanic/Latino
g. Asian/Pacific Islander
h. Native American

New Format NCLEX Questions

1. You are caring for a 21-year-old Hispanic woman admitted to the medical floor where you have your clinical rotation after gashing her leg badly in a car accident. At her bedside is her 30-year-old husband, who is assuming the role of interpreter. The patient understands most English that is spoken to her but can speak very little. She has been able to communicate with you so far that she is in a great deal of pain.

   As the nurse caring for this patient, you recognize that her culture consists of: (*select all that apply*)

   a. Language
   b. Thoughts
   c. Mode of communication
   d. Actions of the patient
   e. Actions of the nurse

f. Customs
g. Belief system
h. Values
i. Institutions unique to racial and ethnic makeup
j. Religious and social groups

2. As you care for this patient, you are trying to maintain an awareness of how her culture can affectr her health behaviors. This most accurately describes ______________.
 a. Acculturation
 b. Assimilation
 c. Inclusion
 d. Diversity
 e. Cultural humility

3. In your clinical rotation, you are working with a Muslim patient who tells you that the patient recently emigrated from her home country and culture and found that her belief system and values were not highly esteemed by the new culture. You recognize that this most accurately describes ______________.
 a. Acculturation
 b. Assimilation
 c. Diversity
 d. Cultural shock
 e. Cultural humility

▶ Case Study

You are caring for a 21-year-old Hispanic woman admitted to the medical floor where you have your clinical rotation after gashing her leg badly in a car accident. At her bedside is her 30-year-old husband, who is assuming the role of interpreter. The patient understands most English that is spoken to her but can speak very little. She has been able to communicate with you so far that she is in a great deal of pain and is concerned about her three children, ages 4, 3, and 6 months.

1. Which part of the scenario above do you view as the greatest barrier to health care for this patient? (*highlight in the paragraph above where the greatest barrier exists*)

Concept Map

Please develop a concept map based on the case study presented above.

Note Taker

I.

II. Characteristics of culture

III. Cultural shock

IV. Functioning as a culture

A. Socialization

B. Acculturation

C. Assimilation

V. Vulnerable populations

VI. Factors affecting communication

References

Baldwin, D. (2003). Disparities in health and health care: Focusing efforts to eliminate unequal burdens. *Online Journal of Issues in Nursing, 8*. www.nursingworld.org/MainMenuCategories/ANAMarketplace/ANAPeriodicals/OJIN/TableofContents/Volume82003/No1Jan2003/DisparitiesinHealthandHealthCare.aspx

Caba, A., & Colon, Y. (Eds). (n.d.). *For health care professionals: Cultural humility in cancer care.* CancerCare. https://media.cancercare.org/publications/original/423-2022_For_Health_Care_Professionals_-_Cultural_Humility_in_Cancer_Care.pdf

Centers for Disease Control and Prevention. (2022). *Leading cause of death, males and females.* https://www.cdc.gov/healthequity/lcod/index.htm.

D'Amico, D., & Barbarito, C. (2015). *Health and physical assessment in nursing* (3rd ed.) Pearson.

Huber, D. (2017). *Leadership and nursing care management* (6th ed.). Elsevier.

Kelly, P., & Tazbir, J. (2013). *Essentials of nursing leadership and management* (3rd ed.). Delmar.

Morello, C., & Keating, D. (2009, September 22). Number of foreign-born U.S. residents drops. *Washington Post.* http://www.washingtonpost.com/wpdyn/content/article/2009/09/21/AR2009092103251.html

Ohlemacher, S. (2007, September 12). 20 percent of people living in U.S. speak language other than English at home. *Post and Courier.* http://www.postandcourier.com/news/2007/sep/12/language15626/

Prasad, S. J., Nair, P., Gadhvi, K., Barai, I., Danish, H. S., & Philip, A. B. (2016, February). Cultural humility: Treating the patient, not the illness. *Medical Education Online, 21*, 30908. doi:10.3402/meo.v21.30908. PMID: 26847853; PMCID: PMC4742464.

Robert Woods Johnson Foundation. (2022). *Achieving health equity.* https://www.rwjf.org/en/library/features/achieving-health-equity.html.

Stanford, F. C. (2020, June). The importance of diversity and inclusion in the healthcare workforce. *Journal of the National Medical Association, 112*(3), 247–249. doi:10.1016/j.jnma.2020.03.014. Epub 2020 Apr 23. PMID: 32336480; PMCID: PMC7387183.

Truman, B., Tinker, T., Vaughan, E., Kapella, B., Brenden, M., Woznica, C., ... Lichveld, M. (2009). Pandemic influenza preparedness and response among immigrants and refugees. *American Journal of Public Health, 99*, S278–S286.

U.S. Department of Health and Human Services. (2022). *Healthy People 2030.* https://health.gov/healthypeople.

Vespa, J., Medina, L., & Armstrong, D. (2020). *Demographic turning points for the United States: Population projections for 2020 to 2060.* https://www.census.gov/library/publications/2020/demo/p25-1144.html.

Wilkinson, J., & Treas, L. (2019). *Fundamentals of nursing* (4th ed.). F. A. Davis.

CHAPTER

7

Informatics

CHAPTER OBJECTIVES

Upon completion of the chapter, you will be able to:

1. Discuss the primary uses of electronic health records
2. Describe the advantages of using telehealth
3. Describe the limitations of using telehealth
4. Describe the anticipated outcomes of use of electronic health records
5. Discuss the three modalities of telehealth
6. Discuss the impact of HIPAA on informatics

KEY TERMS

electronic health record

Health Insurance Portability and Accountability Act of 1996 (HIPAA)

HIPAA Privacy Rule

HIPAA Security Rule

informatics

Health care is a global concern, as was made evident by the COVID19 pandemic, which began in 2020. Subsequently, during the pandemic's duration, nursing has transformed into a global profession as nurses from various countries have provided care to external populations ravaged by the pandemic. This type of global profession requires technology to manage the huge amount of information moving through it. The use of such information technology in health care is **informatics** (Sewell, 2016). It is informatics that will allow you as the nurse to record and review information about multiple patients. It will allow you to provide care to patients that is based on actual data such as laboratory reports and results of procedures (Sewell, 2016).

Informatics has been greatly impacted by the **Health Insurance Portability and Accountability Act of 1996 (HIPAA)**. This legislation provided data privacy and security requirements for safeguarding specific medical information of the public. Significant parts of HIPAA are the **Privacy Rule** and the **Security Rule**. The HIPAA Privacy Rule established national standards to protect the medical records of patients as well as other personal health information. It applies to health plans, health care clearinghouses, as well as any health care providers that utilize electronic health are transactions. While the HIPAA Privacy Rule deals with protected health information (PHI) in general, the HIPAA Security Rule deals specifically with electronic PHI (American Academy of Allergy, Asthma, and Immunology [AAAAI], 2022).

Telehealth

Informatics in the form of telehealth has increased substantially as a result of the COVID19 pandemic. Telehealth is considered to be the exchange of medical information from one site to another using electronic communication in an effort to improve patient health (Tuckson et al., 2017). The Centers for Disease Control and Prevention (CDC; 2020) has noted that telehealth consists of three modalities:

- Synchronous: This would consist of real-time telephone or audio-video interaction with a patient using a computer or a smartphone.
- Asynchronous: This would entail collecting messages, images, or data pertaining to the patient that are interpreted by the provider and then responding to them at a later time.
- Remote: This allows direct transmission of the patient's clinical information from a distance to the health care provider.

The CDC has indicated that telehealth can be used to:

- Access primary care providers for chronic health conditions
- Assist in medication management
- Provide health coaching, nutritional counseling, and assistance in weight management for patients experiencing chronic conditions
- Guide the patient in participating in physical therapy and occupational therapy
- Monitor clinical indicators of chronic medical conditions such as blood pressure
- Provide case management for patients who are having difficulty accessing care such as those who are located in isolated environments or who lack transportation
- Follow up with patients who have been recently hospitalized (see Table 7.1)

TABLE 7.1. Advantages of Telehealth

Instruction	Provide health coaching, nutritional counseling, and assistance in weight management for patients experiencing chronic conditions.
Management	Provide case management for patients who are having difficulty accessing care.
	Assist in medication management.
Access	Access primary care providers for chronic health conditions.
Guidance	Guide the patient in participating in physical therapy and occupational therapy.
Monitor	Monitor clinical indicators of chronic medical conditions.
Follow up	Follow up with patients who have been recently hospitalized.

Changes to HIPAA's Security Rule and its impact on telemedicine were implemented in March 2020 as a result of the COVID19 pandemic. These changes included enforcement discretion on HIPAA violations for use of standard remote communication technologies. The U.S. Department of Health and Human Services' Office for Civil Rights decided to at least temporarily waive penalties for HIPAA violations against health care providers who were serving patients using everyday communication technology such as FaceTime and Skype. This has allowed providers to use nonencrypted platforms such as Apple's FaceTime, Skype, and Zoom for telemedicine purposes. Currently, it remains uncertain if the waivers will remain in effect indefinitely (AAAAI, 2022). The HIPAA guidelines for telemedicine are found within the HIPAA Security Rule and indicate the following:

- Electronic PHI should be accessible only to authorized users.
- The integrity of the electronic PHI must be protected with a system of secure communication.
- Implement a system of monitoring communications containing electronic PHI to prevent breaches of information.

When a medical professional or health care organization creates electronic PHI that will be stored by a third party, the medical professional or health care organization is required to have a Business Associate Agreement with the third party. The Business Associate Agreement must include the methods that will be used by the third party to ensure that the data are protected and there are procedures in place to be utilized for regular auditing of the data's security (AAAAI, 2022).

Never overlook the need for patient consent for telemedicine. Even if your state does not specifically require it, it is a best practice to implement. When developing a consent form for use of telemedicine with a patient, plan to include the following:

- Patient's rights when receiving telemedicine, particularly the right to stop treatment
- Patient's responsibilities when receiving telemedicine, particularly the need to provide accurate and thorough information about symptoms, past illnesses, hospitalizations, medications, and pain
- The formal grievance process to resolve potential ethical concerns that might emerge as a result of telemedicine
- The benefits, constraints, and risks (including privacy and security) of telemedicine
- Telemedicine program policies involving billing, scheduling, and cancellations
- The procedure to utilize should an equipment failure occur during a telemedicine session as well as the contingency plan to follow (AAAAI, 2022)

Patients should always be concerned about their privacy and prepared to question providers regarding how information will be protected during a telemedicine session. Providers should therefore be prepared to educate patients on the process that has been implemented to protect confidential information.

The worldwide impact of telemedicine was revealed during the COVID-19 pandemic. It was seen as a resource that could improve surveillance of patients, curtail the spread of disease, facilitate early identification and management of patients experiencing illness, and guarantee continuity of care of fragile patients who are experiencing multiple chronic diseases.

However, Omboni et al. (2022) noted that there are major issues that still must be addressed to allow telemedicine to be implemented consistently worldwide. These include:

- Establishing sufficient policies to legislate telemedicine, license health care operators, protect the privacy of patients, and implement plans for reimbursement

- Creating and distributing practical guidelines for the routine clinical use of telemedicine in various settings
- Increasing the level of integration of telemedicine with traditional health care delivery
- Improving health care professionals' and patients' awareness of telemedicine as well as increasing their willingness to use it,
- Overcoming inequalities among countries and populations due to barriers in technology, infrastructure, and economies

How can a provider decide if telemedicine is worth the time and money to implement? There are clear benefits to this form of health care delivery. Patients located in rural areas can benefit from receiving both primary and specialty care via telemedicine services. Telemedicine visits can be used for medicine reconciliation, transmission of information from patient monitoring equipment such as glucometers, and management of chronic diseases such as diabetes mellitus, heart failure, and mental health disorders. However, it is important to recognize that telemedicine visits are not a complete substitute for in-person provider visits. There is no opportunity to conduct a hands-on physical examination of the patient or gain an accurate weight of the patient for calculating dosages of weight-based drugs. Also, technical problems and equipment failure can interfere with accurate delivery of health care. Some patients may have limited Internet access or difficulty manipulating equipment due to physical disabilities. As with any deviation from the standard in-person provider visit, the provider should determine whether the patient has sufficient decision-making capacity to give consent for a telemedicine visit (Saljoughian, 2021).

Electronic Health Records

One of the main ways that informatics has affected nursing as a profession is with the development of the electronic health record (EHR). This is an electronic version of a patient's paper chart—a patient-centered record that allows information to be securely accessed by authorized users. According to the Office of the National Coordinator for Health Information Technology (2021), the use of EHRs has resulted in:

- Improved patient care: This has occurred through rapid access to patient records for more coordinated and efficient delivery of care. Documentation has become legible and accurate, thus facilitating hospital reimbursement. Prescribing of medications has subsequently become more reliable as prescriptions have been able to be sent electronically to pharmacies.
- Increased patient participation in care: This has occurred as a result of providers giving patients complete and accurate information about their health. Patients further participate in their care as providers offer follow-up information in the form of discharge instructions, reminders for additional treatments needed, and Internet resources that are available. Patients further participate in their own care through email exchanges with providers. This allows providers to detect significant symptoms early and could possibly prevent patient fatality.

- Improved care coordination: This occurs as patient health information is organized and distributed among all providers involved in patient care. This may prevent medical errors and unnecessary and expensive testing, thus ensuring positive patient care outcomes.
- Improved diagnostics and patient outcomes: This occurs as EHRs allow providers to have reliable and accurate access to a patient's complete medical information. This may allow providers to arrive at a diagnosis earlier. EHRs maintain a thorough record of medications and allergies and thus may prevent possible reactions derived from conflicting medications. EHRs can furthermore improve risk management by providing clinical alerts and reducing opportunities for adverse reactions.
- Practice efficiencies and cost savings: This occurs through a reduction in transcription costs and implementation of error prevention alerts. Billing is more accurate once EHRs are implemented. Patient information is available to providers from any location (see Table 7.2).

TABLE 7.2. Outcomes of Use of Electronic Health Records

ANTICIPATED OUTCOME	DETAILS OF THE OUTCOME
Improved patient care	This has occurred through rapid access to patient records for more coordinated and efficient delivery of care. Documentation has become legible and accurate, thus facilitating hospital reimbursement. Prescribing of medications has become more reliable as prescriptions are sent electronically to pharmacies.
Increased patient participation in care	This has occurred as providers give patients complete and accurate information about their health. Patients further participate in their care as providers offer follow-up discharge instructions, reminders for additional treatments needed, as well as access to Internet resources that are available. Email exchanges with providers allow providers to detect significant symptoms early and could prevent patient fatality.
Improved care coordination	This occurs as patient health information is organized and distributed among all providers involved in patient care. This may prevent medical errors and unnecessary and expensive testing.
Improved diagnostics and patient outcomes	This occurs as EHRs allow providers to have reliable and accurate access to a patient's complete medical information. This may allow providers to arrive at a diagnosis earlier. EHRs maintain a thorough record of medications and allergies and thus may prevent possible reactions derived from conflicting medications. They can furthermore improve risk management by providing clinical alerts and reducing opportunities for adverse reactions.
Practice efficiencies and cost savings	This occurs through a reduction in transcription costs and implementation of error prevention alerts. Billing is more accurate once EHRs are implemented. Patient information is available to providers from any location (Office of the National Coordinator for Health Information Technology, 2020).

As America continues to move slowly through the process of recovering from the effects of the pandemic, both private insurance carriers and some Medicaid providers have become more willing to pay for a telehealth medical appointment, which typically is shorter than an in-person visit and usually foregoes procedures. In addition, some states have relaxed licensing requirements to allow clinicians in one state to conduct telehealth visits with patients in another state. More permissive licensing means that additional guidelines will need to be developed to ensure proper licensing of clinicians (Shachar et al., 2020).

▶ Summary of Key Points in Chapter

This chapter focused on aspects of informatics, including telehealth and EHRs. EHRs were noted to have resulted in improved patient care, improved patient participation in care, improved care coordination, and improved diagnostics and patient outcomes while allowing nurses and health care providers to practice efficiency and control cost savings. Telehealth as a means of exchanging medical information was reviewed. Modalities of telehealth were found to be synchronous, asynchronous, and remote. The multiple purposes of telehealth as enumerated by the CDC were discussed. Finally, the advantages of telehealth were noted to be patient instruction, case management, access to health care, patient guidance, clinical monitoring, and patient follow-up.

▶ Conclusion

A significant part of telehealth is the health teaching that clinicians can provide to patients who are experiencing chronic conditions such as hypertension and diabetes. The teaching-learning process will be discussed in the next chapter.

▶ Critical Thinking Questions

1. Compare and contrast the modalities of telehealth.

2. Think about your own work environment. Provide examples of how use of telehealth can provide advantages in each of the following categories:

    a. Instruction

    b. Management

    c. Access

    d. Guidance

    e. Monitor

    f. Follow-up

3. Your workplace has implemented the use of EHRs. Which outcomes do you anticipate from this implementation?

Scenarios

1. Your facility is planning to implement EHRs during the next fiscal year. You are on the committee that is responsible for selecting the specific software used to implement the health records. The director of your area is concerned that the expense used to implement the new system may overwhelm the facility. What would you tell the director regarding the cost savings that could occur when using an EHR system?

2. Your facility is considering implementing telehealth. The committee that is planning the implementation process intends the telehealth initiative to take place using real-time audio-video interaction with patients using either a computer or a smartphone. Based on this information, which telehealth modality would you anticipate being utilized? Explain your answer.

NCLEX-Style Review Questions

1. Expected outcomes to the implementation of EHRs include: (*select all that apply*)
   a. Improved care coordination
   b. Improved patient care
   c. Decrease in time required for patient care
   d. Increased patient participation in care
   e. Decreased need for diagnostic testing

2. The facility is planning to implement telehealth. It intends to collect patient data that has been interpreted by the provider so that the provider can respond to it at a later time. Which modality will this utilize?
   a. Synchronous
   b. Asynchronous
   c. Remote
   d. Distance

3. The facility is planning to implement telehealth. It intends to allow direct transmission of the patient's clinical information from a distance away to the health care provider within the facility. Which modality will this utilize?
   a. Synchronous
   b. Asynchronous
   c. Remote
   d. Distance

4. The facility is planning to implement telehealth. It intends to allow real-time audio-video interaction with a patient using a computer. Which modality will this utilize?
   a. Synchronous
   b. Asynchronous
   c. Remote
   d. Distance

5. Advantages of telehealth include: (*select all that apply*)
   a. Management
   b. Guidance
   c. Planning
   d. Instruction
   e. Access
   f. Implementation
   g. Monitor
   h. Follow-up
   i. Evaluation

Case Study

You are working on the medical-surgical unit today with Alice. During your break, you begin discussing the facility's expected implementation of telehealth. Alice tells you, "I just don't know that I agree with this decision. I don't see how we can give patients what they need by telehealth rather than by a face-to-face visit. I feel that I can't give a patient what he deserves like this." What would you tell Alice to help her understand how telehealth can be utilized as an effective tool to enhance patient care?

1. According to the CDC, telehealth can be used to: *(select all that apply)*
   a. Access primary care providers for chronic health conditions
   b. Produce significant cost savings
   c. Assist in medication management
   d. Provide health coaching for patients experiencing chronic conditions
   e. Guide the patient in participating in physical therapy and occupational therapy
   f. Monitor clinical indicators of chronic medical conditions
   g. Provide case management for patients who are having difficulty accessing care
   h. Follow up with patients who have been recently hospitalized

2. When developing a consent form for use of telemedicine with a patient, the provider should plan to include: *(select all that apply)*
   a. Patient's rights, particularly the right to stop treatment
   b. Program policies involving billing, scheduling, and cancellations
   c. The formal grievance process to resolve potential ethical concerns
   d. Patient's expected follow-up appointment
   e. The benefits, constraints, and risks, including privacy and security
   f. Patient's responsibilities, particularly the need to provide accurate information
   g. Procedure to utilize if there is an equipment failure and the contingency plan

3. The HIPAA Security Rule deals specifically with ____________.
   a. ____ Protected health information in general
   b. ____health plans and health care clearinghouses
   c. ____electronic protected health information
   d. ____health care providers utilizing electronic care transactions

▶ Concept Map

Create a concept map that describes Alice's situation.

▶ Note Taker

I. Definition of informatics

II. Electronic health records: anticipated outcomes

A. Improved patient care

B. Increased patient participation in care

C. Improved care coordination

D. Improved diagnostics and patient outcomes

E. Practice efficiencies and cost savings

III. Telehealth

A. Modalities

1. Synchronous

2. Asynchronous

3. Remote

B. Advantages

1. Access to primary care provider

2. Assist in medication management

3. Health coaching

4. Patient guidance

5. Monitor clinical indicators

6. Case management

7. Patient follow-up

References

American Academy of Allergy, Asthma, and Immunology. (n.d.). *Security and HIPAA*. https://www.aaaai.org/Allergist-Resources/Telemedicine/HIPAA

Centers for Disease Control and Prevention. (2020). *Using telehealth to expand access to essential health services during the COVID-19 pandemic*. https://www.cdc.gov/coronavirus/2019-ncov/hcp/telehealth.html

Office of the National Coordinator for Health Information Technology. (2021). *Patient Access to Health Records*]. https://www.healthit.gov/topic/patient-access-health-records/patient-access-health-records.

Omboni, S., Padwal, R. S., Alessa, T., Benczúr, B., Green, B. B., Hubbard, I., Kario, K., Khan, N. A., Konradi, A., Logan, A. G., Lu, Y., Mars, M., McManus, R. J., Melville, S., Neumannm, C. L., Paratim, G., Rennam, N. F., Ryvlin, P. ... Wang, J. (2022). The worldwide impact of telemedicine during COVID-19: Current evidence and recommendations for the future. *Connected Health*, *1*, 7–35. doi:10.20517/ch.2021.03

Saljoughian, M. (2021). The benefits and limitations of telehealth. *U.S. Pharmacist*, *46*(8), 5–8.

Sewell, J. (2016). *Informatics and nursing: Opportunities and challenges* (5th ed.). Wolters Kluwer.

Shachar, C., Engel, J., & Elwyn, G. (2020). Implications for telehealth in a postpandemic future: Regulatory and privacy issues. *Journal of the American Medical Association, 323*(23), 2375–2376. doi:10.1001/jama.2020.7943

Tuckson, R. V., Edmunds, M., & Hodgkins, M. L. (2017). Telehealth. *New England Journal of Medicine, 377*(16), 1585–1592. http://dx.doi.org/10.1056/NEJMsr1503323

CHAPTER

8

Teaching-Learning Process

KEY TERMS

affective domain
cognitive domain
psychomotor domain
teaching plan

CHAPTER OBJECTIVES

Upon completion of the chapter, you will be able to:

1. Discuss the various learning domains: affective, cognitive, and psychomotor
2. Describe factors that will affect the learning process
3. Follow the steps of the teaching process
4. Develop a teaching plan that can be implemented

Patient teaching is a significant part of the nurse-patient relationship since trust and respect must exist between the teacher (the nurse) and the learner (the patient and significant others) before learning will occur. The goal of the teaching-learning process is the patient's active participation in health care as the patient complies with the instructions.

Steps in the Teaching-Learning Process

The teaching-learning process consists of the following steps, which are reflective of the nursing process:

1. **Assess the learning needs of the patient:** You'll use all available sources of information to accomplish this objective, including medical records and the completed nursing admission assessment. Determine the overall broad goal for the patient. The patient and family members or significant others will be your best sources of information on the patient's learning needs. Remember to ask the patient's permission to have family members present in teaching sessions. You'll need to identify the knowledge, attitude, or skills that will be needed to be acquired by the patients and/or significant others as well as the domains of learning for these (Brookside Associates, 2007).

   The learning domains will be:

- **Cognitive** involves new information being stored and then recalled
- **Affective** involves changes in attitude, values, or feelings
- **Psychomotor** involves a skill being acquired (Billing & Halstead, 2009)

The learning process will be affected by:

- Patient's developmental level.
- Patient's educational level: If you plan to use written visual aids, determine the patient's reading level. Does the patient speak, read, and write in English?
- Past learning experiences: Adults are able to build current learning upon more past learning than children can.
- Chronological age.
- Physical condition: The patient who is in pain is not prepared to learn anything.
- Sensory abilities: If the patient has a deficit in sight, hearing, or fine motor skills, plan the session to accommodate this. The teaching-learning process cannot occur without communication on the part of both nurse and patient.
- Emotional health: the patient who is anxiously awaiting the results of pending lab tests is not prepared to learn anything.
- Social and economic stability: The patient who is stressed over the need to miss work while hospitalized may not be prepared to undergo a teaching session.
- Motivation to learn: Does the patient want to learn the material? Does the patient view the material as being important and worthy of attention?
- Culture: Does the patient have any cultural beliefs that could contradict the information being presented (DeYoung, 2009)?

Ensure that the patient is ready to learn. This involves much more than physical readiness. Is the patient developmentally ready to acquire the new knowledge or skill? Does the patient have appropriate emotional maturity, motor skills, and intellectual capacity? Remember to assess how much information the patient already has. Identify the strengths of the patient or their significant others. Does the patient have an excellent memory? If you are teaching a patient's family members how to care for the patient in a home setting, find out whether some family members have served as a caregiver before so that there is already an existing knowledge base.

2. **Diagnose the learning needs:** You'll diagnose the deficit when there is a lack of knowledge, attitude, or skill that is hindering the patient's development of their highest possible level of health.
3. **Develop a teaching plan:** For each diagnosed learning need, develop short-term and long-term objectives that are specific and measurable. Choose your teaching strategies. Make certain that your selected strategy is appropriate for the information being taught. For example, if you are teaching a patient how to give themselves injections, you'll need to have a synthetic model available so that the patient can practice the skills needed to administer the injection correctly. Decide how much time will be needed for teaching sessions. It will be more effective to use shorter sessions several times during the day

rather than one lengthy session that tires the patient. Initiate an informal contract with the patient. This will emphasize that although the content is important and the sessions are necessary, you will be there to assist the patient with each aspect of the process. Be positive and enthusiastic about the opportunity.

4. **Implement the teaching plan:** Prepare ahead by gathering any visual aids that you intend to use and by making important notes on 3-in.-by-5-in. cards to help you remember specific points if needed. Start the teaching process by introducing yourself to any family member or significant others who have not met you and who will be present. Make certain that you have prepared a comfortable, well-lit area with privacy for the session. Take cues from the patient to determine if an area needed to be discussed in greater detail.
5. **Evaluate the teaching-learning plan:** Determine if learner objectives have been met. Seek feedback from patients to determine the effectiveness of the teaching. Plan to make some revisions to the teaching-learning plan since there will always be an area that requires refining.

   Determine if the objectives were realistic or were written at too high a level. Was the content at an appropriate level, or was it unrealistic for the learner? Was the time period selected for the teaching sessions appropriate, or should the next session be scheduled on different days and times?
6. **Document the teaching-learning process:** Make certain that you document the diagnosed learning needs of the patient, the broad goal, the specific and measurable objectives, the implementation of the teaching plan, and the evaluation results (Brookside Associates, 2007).

TABLE 8.1. Steps in the Teaching-Learning Process

1. Assess the learning needs of the patient
2. Diagnose learning needs
3. Develop a teaching plan
4. Implement the teaching plan
5. Evaluate the teaching plan
6. Document the teaching-learning process

TABLE 8.2. Factors Affecting the Learning Process

1. Developmental level
2. Educational level
3. Past learning experiences
4. Chronological age
5. Physical condition

(continued on next page)

6. Sensory abilities
7. Emotional health
8. Social and economic stability
9. Motivation to learn
10. Culture

TABLE 8.3. Learning Domains

- **Cognitive:** involves new information being stored and then recalled
- **Affective:** involves changes in attitude, values, or feeling
- **Psychomotor:** involves a skill being acquired

How to Make Your Patient Teaching More Effective

What are some techniques that could be used to make your patient teaching more effective?

- Ask your patient how they learn best and match your teaching style to their learning style. An adult learner may prefer to practice new skills using tactile techniques after they have observed a demonstration. Some learners will want to take notes during the demonstration.
- Allow the patient to handle the equipment to be utilized. If you are working with a diabetic patient, for example, the patient's level of comfort will grow as they manipulate the glucometer and handle the syringes to be used. As their comfort level increases, their skills will also grow.
- As part of the teaching-learning session, practice with the patient enough so that the patient can easily gather needed supplies. Make certain that the patient maintains a list of what is needed each time the procedure is performed in case the patient needs to instruct another caregiver to assist them. Ensure that the patient has an appropriate place to store supplies in their home setting. If the patient travels, make certain that they have an appropriate way to carry supplies with them while away from home. If the patient will need to use special medications (such as insulin), make certain that they are aware of special precautions needed and have these in printed form for the benefit of future caregivers.
- Take your time and plan on multiple sessions. Learning complex skills such as self-catheterization, for example, when a patient is also recovering from illness will be an extensive process that requires a committed and patient instructor. Try to let the patient discover what went wrong if the procedure being practiced goes awry initially. Use encouragement to gently guide the patient while letting them gradually assume greater responsibility for performing the skills unaided. As the patient becomes more adept at performing the procedure, discuss with them situations that might require the procedure to be varied. For example, help them problem-solve what to do if they drop the syringe being used (Younas, 2017).

Summary of Key Points in Chapter

This chapter discussed various aspects of the teaching-learning process as implemented by nurses. Topics covered included:

- Steps in the teaching-learning process
- Assessment of patients' learning needs
- Domains of learning
- Factors affecting the learning process
- Development of a teaching plan
- Utilization of teaching strategies
- Documentation of the teaching-learning process
- Techniques to improve patient teaching

Conclusion

The teaching-learning process is integral to the practice of nursing. All nurses should be prepared to assess the learning needs of patients, determine patients' readiness to learn, develop, implement, and evaluate a teaching plan for a patient based on the identified learning needs, and then document the overall teaching-learning process. The steps of the teaching-learning process are similar to those of the nursing process, which will be discussed in the subsequent chapter.

Critical Thinking Questions

1. Mrs. Smith is a 47-year-old, married mother of three teenagers. She underwent a hysterectomy today as part of the treatment of uterine cancer. She is scheduled to begin chemotherapy in one month. List all of the learning needs of this patient.

2. Compare and contrast the three different domains of learning.

    a. Describe a situation in the teaching-learning process that would involve use of the cognitive domain of learning.

    b. Describe a situation in the teaching-learning process that would involve use of the psychomotor domain of learning.

    c. Describe a situation in the teaching-learning process that would involve use of the affective domain of learning.

3. Which factors do you view as affecting the learning process in the case of Mrs. Smith, whose situation was described in question 1? Be specific as to how each factor that you mention will affect the learning process for Mrs. Smith in her current state.

▶ Scenarios

1. You are developing a teaching plan for Mr. Cole, a 62-year-old man who recently underwent a right below-the-knee amputation after years of poorly controlled diabetes. You are to teach him how to care for his surgical incision once he is discharged. He has always worked as a long-distance truck driver. He is divorced with one adult son who lives in another state.

   a. What are the learning needs for Mr. Cole?

   b. What is the goal for this patient?

   c. Set learner objectives for Mr. Cole.

   d. Which learning domains will be involved in this teaching plan?

   e. Which factors will affect the learning process in Mr. Cole's situation?

   f. How will you determine Mr. Cole's readiness to learn?

g. What do you view as the strengths of Mr. Cole?

h. Describe the teaching strategies that you would use in this case.

i. Describe the teaching session(s). How many sessions will you use? How long will the sessions be? Which visible aids will you utilize?

j. Evaluate the teaching-learning plan for Mr. Cole. How would you determine if learner objectives have been met?

k. How would you determine if the objectives were appropriate for this patient?

l. How would you document the teaching-learning process with Mr. Cole?

NCLEX-Style Review Questions

1. An example of the cognitive learning domain is when:
   a. the patient is able to verbalize the expected side effects of a chemotherapeutic drug and the appropriate treatments to utilize if necessary
   b. the patient changes her attitude about mammograms and decides to schedule one for prevention of breast cancer
   c. the patient is able to successfully complete all the steps involved in urinary self-catheterization
   d. the patient is able to accurately follow the procedure required for a complicated wound dressing on his foot

2. An example of the affective learning domain is when:
   a. a parent accurately verbalizes his child's symptoms of a hypersensitivity reaction to a medication
   b. a parent is able to successfully follow the procedure for administering a tube feeding to her child
   c. a parent changes her mind about not vaccinating her child against diphtheria and decides to schedule an appointment for the vaccine to be administered
   d. a parent is able to successfully administer insulin injections to his child who is a Type 1 diabetic

3. Arrange the steps in the teaching-learning process in the correct order.
   ____ Evaluate the teaching plan
   ____ Develop a teaching plan
   ____ Assess the learning needs of the patient
   ____ Diagnose learning needs
   ____ Implement the teaching plan
   ____ Document the teaching-learning process

Case Study

You are working today on the surgical oncology floor. You are working with Joe, another recent graduate registered nurse. You find Joe looking dejected in the break room at lunchtime. "How are things going for you today?" you ask. "Terrible!" Joe responds. "I've got to find a way to teach Mr. McGee and his family members how to dress his leg wound correctly. He'll receive home health visits twice a week, but the dressings are to be done daily, so he and his wife as well as their teenage children need to be taught how to do this. The problem is that while Mr. McGee is willing to learn, he's scared to death and thinks he can't do it. His wife and kids don't see why they need to know anything about it and think that home health should take care of everything.

They aren't even interested in learning about it. What a mess!" Based on what you know now about the teaching-learning process, what advice can you give to Joe?

1. Based on the scenario, the primary learning domain affecting Mr. McGee's teaching session will be ____________.
   a. a. cognitive
   b. b. affective
   c. c. tactile
   d. d. psychomotor

2. Highlight the area in the scenario that corresponds to the learning domain that will affect Mr. McGee's teaching session (*hot spot question*).

3. Based on the scenario, the primary learning domain affecting Mrs. McGee and the McGee children's teaching session will be ____________.
   a. cognitive
   b. affective
   c. tactile
   d. psychomotor

4. Highlight the area in the scenario that corresponds to the learning domain that will affect Mrs. McGee and the McGee children's teaching session (*hot spot question*).

▶ Concept Map

Create a concept map that describes the current situation with Mr. McGee and his family.

▶ Note Taker

I. Steps in the teaching-learning process

A. Assess the learning needs of the patient

B. Use all sources of information

5. Determine broad goals for the patient

6. Determine learning domains

a. Cognitive

b. Psychomotor

c. Affective

7. Determine readiness to learn

C. Determine learning needs

D. Develop a teaching plan

E. Implement the teaching plan

F. Evaluate the teaching plan

G. Document the teaching plan

II. Factors affecting the learning process

III. Patient's developmental level

A. Patient's educational level

B. Patient's past learning experiences

C. Patient's chronological age

D. Patient's physical condition

E. Patient's sensory abilities

F. Patient's emotional health

G. Patient's social and economic stability

H. Patient's motivation to learn

I. Patient's culture

J. Techniques to improve patient teaching

References

Billings, D., & Halstead, J. (2009). *Teaching in nursing: A guide for faculty* (3rd ed.). Elsevier.

Brookside Associates. (2007). *Nursing fundamentals II multimedia edition—The role of the practical nurse.* Medical Education Division. https://brooksidepress.org/Products/Nursing_Fundamentals_II/lesson_7_Section_1.htm

DeYoung, S. (2009). *Teaching strategies for nurse educators* (2nd ed.). Prentice Hall.

Younas, A. (2017, November/December). The nursing process and patient teaching. *Nursing Made Incredibly Easy!*, *15*(6), 13–16. doi:10.1097/01.NME.0000525549.21786.b5

CHAPTER

9

The Nursing Process

CHAPTER OBJECTIVES

Upon completion of the chapter, you will be able to:

1. Define the nursing process as it is used by the registered nurse
2. Describe the various steps of the nursing process
3. Provide examples of the use of the steps of the nursing process in patient care
4. Describe the various domains of learning as used in Bloom's taxonomy
5. Document examples of the various types of nursing interventions
6. Describe the importance of concept mapping

KEY TERMS

affective domain
assessment
Bloom's taxonomy
concept map
cognitive domain
dependent nursing intervention
domain
emergency assessment
evaluation
focused assessment
independent nursing intervention
initial assessment
interdependent nursing intervention
nursing goal
nursing diagnosis
nursing process
objective data
ongoing assessment
outcome criteria
planning
psychomotor domain
subjective data
taxonomy

Introduction to the Nursing Process

As the registered nurse (RN) functions daily as a nurse leader, they will be called on to exercise critical thinking and nursing judgment. The nurse will be required to demonstrate that they can effectively collect the various pieces of information about a patient's presenting symptoms, existing disease processes, support system, medication regimen, and psychological state to formulate a plan of nursing care for the patient. The process by which those pieces are collected, scrutinized as to their value, and analyzed regarding their applicability to the patient is known as the *nursing process*. Implementation of the nursing process and its subsequent documentation result in the development of a plan for the nursing care of the patient (Gardner, 2002).

Why is the nursing process important? Above all, it is centered around the patient or client. It requires the nurse to individualize the plan being developed, because a generic plan may well serve as an effective framework for a patient but requires specific changes to be made based on the needs of each patient. The nursing process helps the RN (Gardner, 2002):

- Stay organized during collection of data regarding the patient
- Develop a nursing diagnosis to describe the patient's current situation
- Plan a regimen of nursing care to assist in resolving the patient's problem to the greatest extent possible
- Implement the steps involved in the regimen of nursing care
- Evaluate the effectiveness of the care that was carried out

In addition, the nursing process assists the RN in effective use of time management as well as conservation of resources. Those resources may be financial, personnel, or energy. Therefore, the nursing process can lead to effective assessment, so that fewer supplies are charged to the patient; effective planning, so that fewer personnel are required to be assigned to the patient's care; and effective implementation, so that fewer nurses experience physical or emotional exhaustion in caring for a chronically ill patient.

The advantages of the nursing process when used effectively are as follows (Alfaro-Lefevre, 2009):

- To ensure the patient's health concerns and their response to them are the focus of the nursing care plan
- To ensure care that is planned and implemented is individualized for the patient
- To promote the patient's participation in their care by encouraging autonomy as the plan is implemented, and to provide the patient with a sense of control rather than the helplessness that can come with long-term assumption of the patient role
- To improve communication by providing nurses with a summary of the patient's identified health issues and all current data known about the issues
- To require accountability for nursing actions that are implemented; such accountability then promotes delivery of the highest-quality health care
- To require the use of critical thinking, problem-solving, and nursing judgment
- To focus on the achievement of patient outcomes
- To minimize errors that can occur during the delivery of patient care

Assessment

Assessment is arguably the most important step in the nursing process because it involves data collection on the various health issues being experienced by the patient.

Both licensed practical nurses and RNs can contribute to data collection, but only the RN analyzes the data and uses them to formulate a comprehensive assessment of the patient that will ultimately be used in the development of a plan of nursing care (Quan, 2007).

For an assessment to be comprehensive, it must be holistic, and this can only occur if the data gathered include a physical examination and an exhaustive health history. The data gathered through the health history should include subjective data, or information retrieved from the patient's verbalization, and objective data, or information retrieved from observation of the patient, including reviewing the results of diagnostic testing. The data gathered through assessment can occur through four variations of this process (Table 9.1):

1. **Initial assessment:** This occurs on initial contact with the patient and is usually as comprehensive as possible. It begins with the symptoms that caused the patient to seek assistance from the health care community and should culminate in a head-to-toe view of the patient's level of functioning (Harkreader et al., 2007).
2. **Focused assessment:** This is performed on each problem once identified. This type of assessment is important because it allows symptoms to be examined in greater detail, promotes the weighing of various etiologies to explain those symptoms, searches for contributing factors, and examines patient characteristics that would also help solve the presenting problem or at least clarify the issue. Focused assessment will be initiated again if a new symptom or problem suddenly emerges.
3. **Emergency assessment:** This is used when time is of the essence due to the life-threatening nature of the patient's problem. It includes only essential data relevant to the patient's immediate issue. Once the patient's situation is stable and is no longer considered life-threatening, additional data can be gathered (Harkreader et al., 2007).
4. **Ongoing assessment:** This occurs continuously throughout a patient's health care experience. Data may be gathered with the assistance of electronic equipment, and the ongoing assessment usually includes periodic episodes of routine data gathering, such as every four hours for vital signs. The interval for such ongoing assessment may change at the discretion of the RN, in some cases (Harkreader et al., 2007).

TABLE 9.1. Types of Assessment

TYPE OF NURSING ASSESSMENT	CHARACTERISTICS
Initial	This occurs upon initial contact with the patient and is as comprehensive as possible. It begins with the symptoms that caused the patient to seek assistance from the healthcare community and should result in a head-to-toe view of the patient's level of functioning.
Focused	The focused assessment is performed on each problem that has been identified. This type of assessment allows symptoms to be examined in greater detail, promotes the weighing of etiologies to explain the symptoms, searches for contributing factors, and examines patient characteristics that would also help solve the presenting problem or at least clarify the issue. Focused assessment will be initiated again if a new symptom or problem suddenly emerges.
Emergency	This is utilized when time is of the essence due to the life-threatening nature of the patient's problem. It will include only essential data that is relevant to the patient's immediate issue. Once the patient's situation is stable and is no longer considered life-threatening, additional data can be gathered.

TYPE OF NURSING ASSESSMENT	CHARACTERISTICS
Ongoing	This is considered to be occurring continuously throughout a patient's healthcare experience. Data may be gathered with the assistance of electronic equipment such as may be seen in a critical care unit, and the ongoing assessment usually will include periodic episodes of data-gathering that occur routinely, such as every four hours for vital signs, for example. The interval for such ongoing assessment may be able to be changed at the discretion of the RN, in some cases.

As the RN begins the process of analyzing the data, they will find that it can be classified as either subjective or objective. **Subjective data** are pieces of information received from the patient because they cannot be observed directly by the nurse. Examples of subjective data include pain, nausea, and dizziness. In comparison, **objective data** are considered to be pieces of information about the client obtained through direct observation. This type of data yields information that is measurable. Examples of objective data are blood pressure, pulse, respiration, and temperature readings (Harkreader et al., 2007).

The data comprising the assessment phase of the nursing process can be gathered through physical examination of the patient, observation of the characteristics of the patient's symptoms, review of the results of laboratory and diagnostic tests, discussion with other health professionals, and, most importantly, through interviewing the patient. Such an interview should focus on the patient's chief complaint that led them to seek medical assistance and should include a discussion of the patient's past medical history; family medical history' and pertinent religious, cultural, and psychosocial concerns. The interview should include a summary of the important information gleaned from the discussion with the patient (Harkreader et al., 2007).

Diagnosis

Once assessment information has been gathered and analyzed and the RN has begun making decisions about patient care, a nursing diagnosis can be selected. The **nursing diagnosis** is both measurable and realistic and is used to direct the nursing process as it is individualized for the patient. A list of accepted nursing diagnoses was developed by the North American Nursing Diagnosis Association (NANDA, 2011). These diagnoses are classified using a system known as ***taxonomy***. The classification system yields 13 domains that are then subdivided into classes and, ultimately, into diagnoses (NANDA, 2011). The domains are as follows:

- Activity/rest
- Circulation
- Ego integrity
- Elimination
- Food/fluid
- Hygiene
- Neurosensory
- Pain/discomfort

- Respiration
- Safety
- Sexuality
- Social interaction
- Teaching/learning

Table 9.2 shows the nursing diagnoses developed by NANDA according to the respective domain.

TABLE 9.2. Approved NANDA Nursing Diagnosis List 2018–2020

NANDA Nursing Diagnosis
Domain 1. Health promotion
Class 1. Health awareness
Decreased diversional activity engagement (Nursing Care Plan) Readiness for enhanced health literacy Sedentary lifestyle (Nursing Care Plan)
Class 2. Health management
Frail elderly syndrome (Nursing Care Plan) Risk for frail elderly syndrome Deficient community health Risk-prone health behavior Ineffective health maintenance (Nursing Care Plan) Ineffective health management Readiness for enhanced health management Ineffective family health management Ineffective protection
NANDA Nursing Diagnosis
Domain 2. Nutrition
Class 1. Ingestion
Imbalanced nutrition: less than body requirements (Nursing Care Plan) Readiness for enhanced nutrition Insufficient breast milk production Ineffective breastfeeding (Nursing Care Plan) Interrupted breastfeeding (Nursing Care Plan) Readiness for enhanced breastfeeding Ineffective adolescent eating dynamics Ineffective child-eating dynamics Ineffective infant-feeding dynamics Ineffective infant-feeding pattern (Nursing Care Plan) Obesity Overweight Risk for overweight Impaired swallowing (Nursing Care Plan)

Class 2. Digestion
This class does not currently contain any diagnoses
Class 3. Absorption
This class does not currently contain any diagnoses
Class 4. Metabolism
Risk for unstable blood glucose level (Nursing Care Plan) Neonatal hyperbilirubinemia Risk for neonatal hyperbilirubinemia Risk for impaired liver function Risk for metabolic imbalance syndrome
Class 5. Hydration
Risk for electrolyte imbalance Risk for imbalanced fluid volume Deficient fluid volume (Nursing Care Plan) Risk for deficient fluid volume Excess fluid volume (Nursing Care Plan)
NANDA Nursing Diagnosis
Domain 3. Elimination and exchange
Class 1. Urinary function
Impaired urinary elimination Functional urinary incontinence Overflow urinary incontinence Reflex urinary incontinence Stress urinary incontinence Urge urinary incontinence Risk for urge urinary incontinence Urinary retention
Class 2. Gastrointestinal function
Constipation (Nursing Care Plan) Risk for constipation Perceived constipation Chronic functional constipation Risk for chronic functional constipation Diarrhea Dysfunctional gastrointestinal motility Risk for dysfunctional gastrointestinal motility Bowel incontinence
Class 3. Integumentary function
This class does not currently contain any diagnoses
Class 4. Respiratory function

(continued on next page)

Impaired gas exchange

NANDA Nursing Diagnosis

Domain 4. Activity/Rest

Class 1. Sleep/Rest

Insomnia
Sleep deprivation
Readiness for enhanced sleep
Disturbed sleep pattern

Class 2. Activity/Exercise

Risk for disuse syndrome
Impaired bed mobility
Impaired physical mobility
Impaired wheelchair mobility
Impaired sitting
Impaired standing
Impaired transfer ability
Impaired walking

Class 3. Energy Balance

Imbalanced energy field
Fatigue
Wandering

Class 4. Cardiovascular/Cardiopulmonary Responses

Activity intolerance
Risk for activity intolerance
Ineffective breathing pattern
Decreased cardiac output
Risk for decreased cardiac output
Impaired spontaneous ventilation
Risk for unstable blood pressure
Risk for decreased cardiac tissue perfusion
Risk for ineffective cerebral tissue perfusion
Ineffective peripheral tissue perfusion
Risk for ineffective peripheral tissue perfusion
Dysfunctional ventilatory weaning response

Class 5. Self-Care

Impaired home maintenance
Bathing self-care deficit
Dressing self-care deficit
Feeding self-care deficit
Toileting self-care deficit
Readiness for enhanced self-care
Self-neglect

NANDA Nursing Diagnosis

Domain 5. Perception/Cognition

Class 1. Attention

Unilateral neglect

Class 2. Orientation

This class does not currently contain any diagnoses

Class 3. Sensation/perception

This class does not currently contain any diagnoses

Class 4. Cognition

Acute confusion
Risk for acute confusion
Chronic confusion
Labile emotional control
Ineffective impulse control
Deficient knowledge
Readiness for enhanced knowledge
Impaired memory

Class 5. Communication

Readiness for enhanced communication
Impaired verbal communication

NANDA Nursing Diagnosis

Domain 6. Self-perception

Class 1. Self-concept

Hopelessness
Readiness for enhanced hope
Risk for compromised human dignity
Disturbed personal identity
Risk for disturbed personal identity
Readiness for enhanced self-concept

Class 2. Self-Esteem

Chronic low self-esteem
Risk for chronic low self-esteem
Situational low self-esteem
Risk for situational low self-esteem

Class 3. Body Image

Disturbed body image

NANDA Nursing Diagnosis

Domain 7. Role Relationship

(continued on next page)

Class 1. Caregiving Roles

Caregiver role strain
Risk for caregiver role strain
Impaired parenting
Risk for impaired parenting
Readiness for enhanced parenting

Class 2. Family Relationships

Risk for impaired attachment
Dysfunctional family processes
Interrupted family processes
Readiness for enhanced family processes

Class 3. Role Performance

Ineffective relationship
Risk for ineffective relationship
Readiness for enhanced relationship
Parental role conflict
Ineffective role performance
Impaired social interaction

NANDA Nursing Diagnosis

Domain 8. Sexuality

Class 1. Sexual Identity

This class does not currently contain any diagnoses

Class 2. Sexual Function

Sexual dysfunction
Ineffective sexuality pattern

Class 3. Reproduction

Ineffective childbearing process
Risk for ineffective childbearing process
Readiness for enhanced childbearing process
Risk for disturbed maternal-fetal dyad

NANDA Nursing Diagnosis

Domain 9. Coping/Stress Tolerance

Class 1. Post-Trauma Responses

Risk for complicated immigration transition
Post-trauma syndrome
Risk for post-trauma syndrome
Rape-trauma syndrome
Relocation stress syndrome
Risk for relocation stress syndrome

Class 2. Coping Responses

Ineffective activity planning
Risk for ineffective activity planning
Anxiety (Nursing Care Plan)
Defensive coping
Ineffective coping
Readiness for enhanced coping
Ineffective community coping
Readiness for enhanced community coping
Compromised family coping
Disabled family coping
Readiness for enhanced family coping
Death anxiety
Ineffective denial
Fear
Grieving
Complicated grieving
Risk for complicated grieving
Impaired mood regulation
Powerlessness
Risk for powerlessness
Readiness for enhanced power
Impaired resilience
Risk for impaired resilience
Readiness for enhanced resilience
Chronic sorrow
Stress overload

Class 3. Neurobehavioral Stress

Acute substance withdrawal syndrome
Risk for acute substance withdrawal syndrome
Autonomic dysreflexia
Risk for autonomic dysreflexia
Decreased intracranial adaptive capacity
Neonatal abstinence syndrome
Disorganized infant behavior
Risk for disorganized infant behavior
Readiness for enhanced organized infant behavior

NANDA Nursing Diagnosis

Domain 10. Life Principles

Class 1. Values

This class does not currently contain any diagnoses

Class 2. Beliefs

Readiness for enhanced spiritual well-being

Class 3. Value/Belief/Action Congruence

(continued on next page)

Readiness for enhanced decision-making
Decisional conflict
Impaired emancipated decision-making
Risk for impaired emancipated decision-making
Readiness for enhanced emancipated decision-making
Moral distress
Impaired religiosity
Risk for impaired religiosity
Readiness for enhanced religiosity
Spiritual distress
Risk for spiritual distress

NANDA Nursing Diagnosis

Domain 11. Safety/Protection

Class 1. Infection

Risk for infection
Risk for surgical site infection

Class 2. Physical Injury

Ineffective airway clearance
Risk for aspiration
Risk for bleeding (Nursing Care Plan)
Impaired dentition
Risk for dry eye
Risk for dry mouth
Risk for falls
Risk for corneal injury
Risk for injury
Risk for urinary tract injury
Risk for perioperative positioning injury
Risk for thermal injury
Impaired oral mucous membrane integrity
Risk for impaired oral mucous membrane integrity
Risk for peripheral neurovascular dysfunction
Risk for physical trauma
Risk for vascular trauma
Risk for pressure ulcer
Risk for shock
Impaired skin integrity (Nursing Care Plan)
Risk for impaired skin integrity
Risk for sudden infant death
Risk for suffocation
Delayed surgical recovery
Risk for delayed surgical recovery
Impaired tissue integrity
Risk for impaired tissue integrity
Risk for venous thromboembolism

Class 3. Violence

Risk for female genital mutilation
Risk for other-directed violence
Risk for self-directed violence
Self-mutilation
Risk for self-mutilation
Risk for suicide

Class 4. Environmental Hazards

Contamination
Risk for contamination
Risk for occupational injury
Risk for poisoning

Class 5. Defensive Processes

Risk for adverse reaction to iodinated contrast media
Risk for allergy reaction
Latex allergy reaction
Risk for latex allergy reaction

Class 6. Thermoregulation

Hyperthermia
Hypothermia
Risk for hypothermia
Risk for perioperative hypothermia
Ineffective thermoregulation
Risk for ineffective thermoregulation

NANDA Nursing Diagnosis

Domain 12. Comfort

Class 1. Physical Comfort

Impaired comfort
Readiness for enhanced comfort
Nausea
Acute pain
Chronic pain
Chronic pain syndrome
Labor pain

Class 2. Environmental Comfort

Impaired comfort
Readiness for enhanced comfort

Class 3. Social Comfort

Impaired comfort
Readiness for enhanced comfort
Risk for loneliness
Social isolation

(continued on next page)

NANDA Nursing Diagnosis
Domain 13. Growth/Development
Class 1. Growth
This class does not currently contain any diagnoses
Class 2. Development
Risk for delayed development

Source: North American Nursing Diagnosis Association. (*n.d.*). Approved NANDA nursing diagnosis list 2018–2020. *https://ar.israa.edu.ps/uploads/documents/2020/02/4gcMo.pdf*

How is a nursing diagnosis formulated? The diagnosis consists of a problem combined with a primary cause, also referred to as the *etiology*, if such information is known. Five types of problems may be experienced by the patient (Gardner, 2002; Table 9.3):

Actual:: This problem is currently experienced by the patient

- Can be validated by specific symptoms the patient notices along with specific signs observed by the nurse
- When combined with a contributing cause, an example of a nursing diagnosis of this type is: Self-care deficit related to bilateral forearm casts

Risk: This problem could develop in the future because of the presence of specific risk factors

- Is almost inevitable unless nursing measures are implemented to stop the progression of the risk factors
- Is validated by the presence of the risk factors
- When combined with a contributing cause, an example of a nursing diagnosis of this type is: Risk for impairment of skin integrity related to inability to get out of bed without assistance

Possible: This problem could develop if additional risk factors develop but will not develop until enough risk factors are present to change this diagnosis to a "risk" problem

- When combined with a contributing cause, an example of a nursing diagnosis of this type is: Possible fluid volume deficit related to occasional nausea

Wellness: This is a progression from one level of wellness to a higher level of wellness

- Cannot be used unless the patient has indicated a desire for a greater level of wellness and the level of functioning on the patient's part must be already effective
- Because the client is already healthy for this diagnosis to be used, no etiology is included because there is no problem
- An example of a nursing diagnosis of this type is: Readiness for enhanced therapeutic regimen management

Syndrome: This diagnosis includes a group of nursing diagnoses that all relate to a specific situation

- Indicates that a serious clinical situation has developed
- Usually there is no etiology present because the use of a syndrome diagnosis
- indicates the contributing factors in the diagnosis
- An example of a nursing diagnosis of this type is: Relocation stress syndrome

TABLE 9.3. Types of Nursing Problems

TYPE OF PROBLEM	DESCRIPTION OF PROBLEM	EXAMPLE OF NURSING DIAGNOSIS
Actual	This is a problem that is being experienced by the patient currently and can be validated by specific symptoms that he or she notices, along with specific signs that can be observed by the nurse.	Self-care deficit related to bilateral forearm casts
Risk	This is a problem that could develop in the future because of the presence of specific risk factors. The problem is almost inevitable unless nursing measures are implemented to stop the progression of the risk factors. The presence of the risk factors validates the diagnosis.	Risk for impairment of skin integrity related to inability to get out of bed without assistance
Possible	This is a problem that could develop if additional risk factors develop. Currently, not enough risk factors are present to change this diagnosis to a "risk" problem.	Possible fluid volume deficit related to occasional nausea
Wellness	This is a progression from one level of wellness to a higher level of wellness. The patient must have indicated that there is a desire for a greater level of wellness, and the level of functioning on the patient's part must be already effective. Since the client is already healthy for this diagnosis to be utilized, no etiology is included because there is no problem.	Readiness for enhanced therapeutic regimen management
Syndrome	This diagnosis includes a group of nursing diagnoses that all relate to a specific situation. The purpose of the diagnosis is to indicate that there is a serious clinical situation that has developed. Usually there is no etiology present since the use of a syndrome diagnosis indicates	Relocation stress syndrome

Wilkinson (2011) stressed the importance of using the process of formulating a nursing diagnosis to help the RN progress in thinking critically. This process of selecting appropriate nursing diagnoses can assist the RN in developing the skill of evaluating a patient's current situation and accurately judging the diagnoses applicable and the nursing interventions that will most effectively assist the patient. Wilkinson (2011) recommended the following questions for the nurse who is determining a nursing diagnosis:

- What actual problems did I identify during assessment of the patient?
- What could be the possible causes of these problems?
- Is this patient at risk of developing other problems?
- If the patient is at risk of developing other problems, what factors are involved in making them subject to doing so?
- Did the patient express a desire to develop a higher level of wellness in their life?

The relationship of these questions to the process of formulating nursing diagnoses is summarized in Figure 9.1.

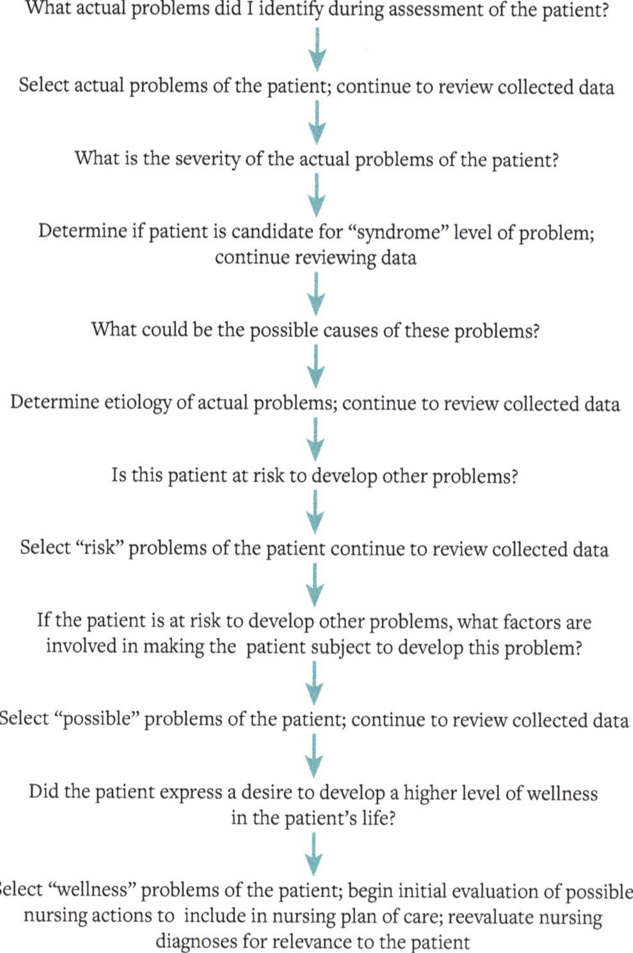

FIGURE 9.1. Critical Thinking Questions to Ask When Formulating Nursing Diagnoses

A third element can be included in the nursing diagnosis to further individualize it to the characteristics of the patient, that is, the signs and symptoms the RN observes in the patient. NANDA refers to the inclusion of these factors as the "defining characteristics" of the patient's nursing diagnosis. The phrase *as evidenced by* can be included to make the diagnosis more specific to the patient's situation.

Using the nursing diagnosis of "Self-care deficit related to bilateral forearm casts" shown in Table 9.2, an example of how this could be used follows. If signs and symptoms the nurse observed that clearly indicated a self-care deficit was present were included, the diagnosis could be changed to read "Self-care deficit related to bilateral forearm casts as evidenced inability to feed self or comb hair." Such defining characteristics often are easier to add to an existing diagnosis after caring for a patient for at least an entire shift so that more lengthy observation is possible and a relationship can be established. Some experts advise using the phrase "secondary to" with a nursing diagnosis to specify the medical condition of the patient as part of the etiology (an example is "Self-care deficit related to bilateral forearm casts secondary to osteomyelitis"), but such phrasing should be used with caution, because it is all too easy to result in a medical diagnosis rather than a nursing diagnosis (Chitty & Black, 2007).

Planning

Once all applicable nursing diagnoses have been selected, the **planning** phase of the nursing process begins. In this phase the RN prioritizes the diagnoses based on the immediate needs of the patient, such as airway, breathing, and circulation. The RN collaborates with the patient to design goals to determine the choice of nursing interventions to assist the patient in resolution of the problem and also to indicate the amount of progress that is being made (Chitty & Black, 2007).

Goals are typically written to center around one of three **domains**, or categories, of learning as indicated in **Bloom's taxonomy**. Bloom was an educator who determined that learning occurred according to three basic categories of activities: **psychomotor**, **cognitive**, and **affective**. The psychomotor domain involves physical movement, and thus learning in this category can be assessed according to distance, time, and speed. The following is an example of a **nursing goal** written using this domain: "Patient will ambulate 12 feet three times daily with assistance." In comparison, the cognitive domain involves knowledge and intellectual skill. An example of a nursing goal written using this domain is "Patient will describe three signs of infection in her surgical incision by date of discharge." Finally, the affective domain involves feelings, values, and attitudes, and therefore an example of a nursing goal written using this domain is "Patient will report feeling accepting of her mastectomy surgical site by date of discharge" (Chitty & Black, 2007).

Both short-term and long-term goals should be developed, with short-term goals being achieved within hours or days and long-term goals requiring a lengthier period of time to be achieved. It is not unheard of for a long-term goal to require months to be accomplished, because it frequently can pertain to rehabilitation (Chitty & Black, 2007).

Goals can be made measurable through the development of **outcome criteria**. Outcome criteria specify the terms under which the goal will be met. Each goal can have several outcome criteria. Outcome criteria describe the conditions under which the patient will act to accomplish the goal and ultimately solve the problem and therefore are indicated by the phrase *as evidenced by* written after the goal. For example, if the goal is "Patient will report feeling accepting of her mastectomy surgical site by date of discharge," the accompanying outcome criteria would be incorporated into the goal as "Patient will report feeling accepting of her mastectomy surgical site by date of discharge as evidenced by (1) asking to view site by postoperative day 3 and (2) asking to perform dressing change without assistance by date of discharge" (Chitty & Black, 2007). If the goal and outcome criteria are written correctly, they should give a clear indication of the nursing interventions needed to assist in the accomplishment of the goals.

Intervention

Both short-term and long-term goals are written during the planning stage of the nursing process. These are particularly important because, along with the outcome criteria that make them measurable, they indicate the nursing orders that dictate the nursing interventions needed to fulfill the goals. Each goal will have its own set of nursing orders, such as "Instruct on dressing change procedure prior to discharge" (Chitty & Black, 2007).

There are three basic types of nursing interventions: dependent, independent, and interdependent (Table 9.4). **Dependent nursing interventions** require supervision from another health care professional, such as a physician or a nurse practitioner. The supervision is necessary because the intervention requires an order for an action that is outside the scope of practice for the RN. For example, medication administration requires that an initial order is written by a physician or a nurse practitioner who has prescribing privileges that cover the substance being ordered.

TABLE 9.4. Types of Nursing Interventions

TYPE OF INTERVENTION	DESCRIPTION	EXAMPLE
Dependent	Requires supervision from another health care professional, such as a physician or a nurse practitioner. The supervision is necessary because the intervention will require an order for an action that is outside the scope of practice for the registered nurse.	Administration of a medication will require an initial order to be written by a physician or nurse practitioner.
Independent	Requires no supervision from personnel other than the registered nurse. The nurse will have all necessary information and skill needed to implement them.	Observe the patient's urine hourly for color and clarity.
Interdependent	Requires collaboration and consultation with other health care professionals during the implementation of the action. Direct supervision from the other health care professional is not required because the intervention is not one that is necessarily outside of the RN's scope of practice, but consultation is required because the other professional has expertise that the RN usually does not possess.	Nursing order is written for an intervention involving a specific type of breathing exercise with which the RN is only vaguely familiar. The assistance of the facility's respiratory therapist will be required.

In comparison, independent nursing interventions are those that require no supervision from personnel other than the RN. The nurse will have all necessary information and skill needed to implement them. An example of an intervention could be to observe the patient's urine hourly for color and clarity. Most types of nursing interventions that involve teaching are usually independent unless they involve instruction on specific areas of expertise that are unfamiliar to the RN or are outside of their scope of practice (Chitty & Black, 2007).

Finally, interdependent nursing interventions require collaboration and consultation with other health care professionals during the implementation of the action. Direct supervision from another health care professional is not required because the intervention is not one that is necessarily outside of the RN's scope of practice, but consultation is required because the other professional has expertise the RN usually does not possess. For example, this could be required if a nursing order is written for an intervention involving a specific type of breathing exercise with which the RN is only vaguely familiar. Thus, the RN would develop an interdependent nursing intervention requiring the assistance of the facility's respiratory therapist (Chitty & Black, 2007).

As nursing orders are written and nursing interventions are developed, it is very important to remember that the interventions must be both patient-centered and related to a specific goal. This means the intervention clearly provides for individualized care for the patient based on their current health status in its comprehensive state, both physical and psychosocial, and also considering their knowledge needs (Alfaro-Lefevre, 2009).

When considering the various needs of the patient in preparation for writing nursing interventions, it may be helpful to review Maslow's Hierarchy of Needs. Maslow was a psychologist who proposed that humans are motivated by basic needs, with some of the most basic needs requiring satisfaction before some of the higher level needs can be addressed and satisfied. This means a person who lacks adequate shelter and food must have these basic needs satisfied before they can address the need for a stable, intimate relationship (Chitty & Black, 2007). Maslow's hierarchy is described in detail in Figure 9.2.

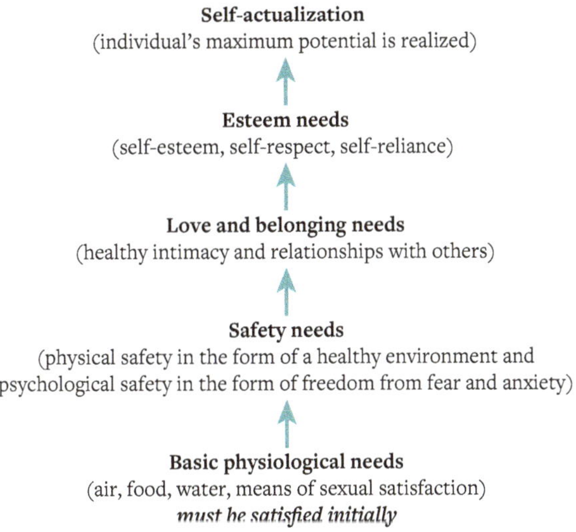

FIGURE 9.2. Maslow's Hierarchy of Needs

Evaluation

Once nursing orders have been written and nursing interventions developed and implemented, the RN can progress forward into the final stage of the nursing process. Gardner (2002) noted that it is during the evaluation stage when the RN decides whether the goals they developed in collaboration with the patient were actually fulfilled. When the goals were either not fulfilled or only partially fulfilled, the RN should gather additional data through reassessment, critically scrutinize the nursing diagnosis to determine if it is still valid, and possibly shelve it in favor of a diagnosis that is now more appropriate for the patient (Gardner, 2002). The RN can determine if goals were met by measuring the expected outcomes of the nursing interventions against the actual outcomes. Subsequently, the RN should record the outcomes as being met, unmet, or partially met (Harkreader et al., 2007). For example, if the patient goal is to experience a manageable level of discomfort as evidenced by the outcome criteria of reporting a pain level no greater than 5 on a 1- to 10-point scale and showing no signs or symptoms of discomfort such as grimacing, perspiring, and moaning, then the RN should determine if the goal was met by examining the outcome criteria. If the patient reports a level of discomfort of 4 on a 1 to 10-point scale but does demonstrate occasional grimacing, then the RN should record the goal in this case as being partially met.

When the RN determines the goal was either not met or was partially met, they must also determine possible reasons for the client's lack of progress toward fulfillment of the goal. Failure to achieve the goal can usually be traced to the following (Alfaro-Lefevre, 2009):

- The nursing diagnosis used to develop the goal was not accurate.
- The goal was not realistic for the patient based on their abilities.
- The nursing interventions were inappropriate for achieving the outcome criteria.
- The patient's medical orders changed and thus invalidated the goal.

Concept Mapping

A variation on the nursing process is the concept map. It is a way of visualizing a patient situation while also integrating theory with practice. Typically, the concept map places patient information in the center of the page and adds additional information such as the patient's diagnosis, diagnostic data, interventions, and treatment goals. Each of these will be represented by different shapes. Relationships will be drawn using solid lines with arrows connecting the concepts (Luchowski, 2003). An example of a concept map is included in Figure 9.3. In the sample concept map, patient admitting information is provided in the rectangle, patient assessment information is noted in the triangles, and nursing interventions are found in the circles. The map could easily be expanded to include collaborative interventions and nursing diagnoses as well.

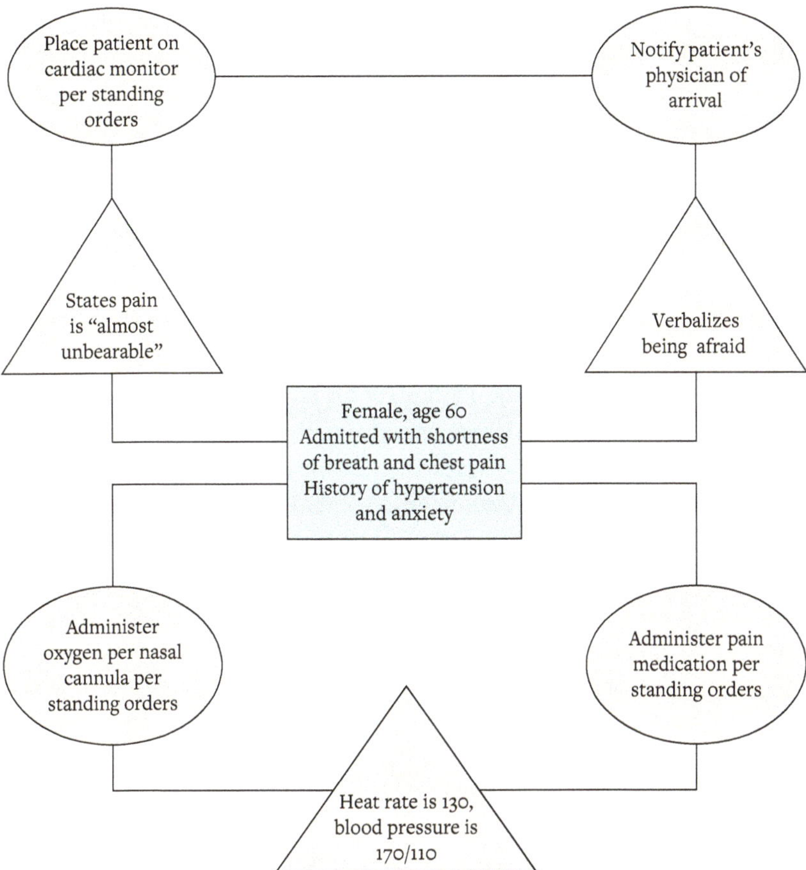

FIGURE 9.3. Example of a Concept Map

▶ Summary of Key Points in Chapter

The chapter described the RN's use of the nursing process in patient care. The various stages of the nursing process were reviewed: assessment, diagnosis, planning, implementation, and evaluation. The specific types of assessment were discussed, such as:

- Initial assessment
- Emergency assessment
- Focused assessment
- Ongoing assessment

In addition, the mechanics of formulating nursing diagnoses as well as writing goals and outcome criteria were discussed, including:

- Using the domains of learning as described in Bloom's taxonomy: affective, cognitive, and psychomotor
- Differentiating between subjective and objective data

- Formulating outcome criteria so that they are measurable and specific
- Differentiating between dependent, independent, and interdependent nursing interventions
- Clearly tying the outcome criteria back to the goal

Finally, the importance of concept mapping was discussed and a sample concept map was included.

Conclusion

A primary responsibility of the RN is to create an organized plan of nursing care for the patient. The plan can only be designed within the confines of the nursing process to ensure it leads to continuity of nursing care and other health care provided in the current health care delivery system.

The stages of the nursing process—assessment, diagnosis, planning, implementation, and evaluation—fit together like puzzle pieces to create a plan to make inpatient care of the highest quality as well as discharge and home care follow-up priorities for the nurse and patient.

Assessment and the data collection that comprise this stage of the process are the most important parts of the entire nursing process. Part of data collection is the research needed to achieve a sufficient understanding of the patient's current health condition. We continue our data collection in the next chapter by discussing the nursing theory.

Critical Thinking Questions

1. Discuss the four types of nursing assessment and describe when it is most appropriate in your nursing practice as an RN to use each type.

    a. What type of information could you obtain using each type of nursing assessment?

2. You are caring for Mr. Smith, a patient who was just admitted to the medical-surgical floor complaining of persistent left upper quadrant abdominal pain. Describe how you might be required to use each of the four types of nursing assessment during your care of Mr. Smith during a 12-hour shift.

3. You are the nurse manager of a nursing unit that is attempting to be more thorough in its documentation of the daily use of the nursing process. One of the personnel that you recently hired is a new graduate licensed practical nurse who is uncertain as to how the nursing process should be used in his daily patient care. Explain in simplified terms how he should be expected to use the nursing process daily.

4. In your job as a nurse manager, you find the hospital education department has just purchased some computer software that will generate nursing diagnoses based on the input of some basic information. You overhear one of the new nurses express relief that "now we have premade diagnoses, and we don't have to figure out how they can be individualized!" Explain how you would intervene to counsel this nurse on the importance of individualizing nursing diagnoses to the specific patient.

Scenarios

1. You are caring for Mr. Jones, a 52-year-old man who drove himself to the emergency department and presented complaining of persistent chest pain and pressure. He smokes one pack of cigarettes daily, is morbidly obese, and reports being severely stressed at his job as an accountant. His wife is a pharmaceutical representative who travels approximately four days per week. Together, they have two teenage boys. Assess this situation thoroughly and try to identify all possible nursing diagnoses. When you identify a nursing diagnosis, also identify an etiology for it as well as defining characteristics, if you believe this will strengthen the diagnosis.

    a. Review scenario 1. Prioritize the nursing diagnoses, select the top three, and write a goal with outcome criteria for each diagnosis. Also, write at least one long-term goal.

    b. Review the domains of learning that are part of Bloom's taxonomy. Use the nursing diagnoses you wrote in scenario 2 and write a goal for each diagnosis that will pertain to each domain of learning. When you finish, each diagnosis should have a goal in the psychomotor domain, a goal in the cognitive domain, and a goal in the affective domain.

2. You are caring for Mrs. Smith, a 58-year-old woman who underwent a mastectomy three days ago. She is scheduled to begin chemotherapy treatments for stage 3 breast cancer in four weeks. She is divorced with one 21-year-old daughter who is in college in another state. You find Mrs. Smith crying one morning when you come in to assess her at the beginning of your shift. She tells you, "I am so afraid to look at my wound. I feel so ugly!"

    a. Assess Mrs. Smith and write down all the pertinent pieces of information you identify from this scenario. Identify the information as either subjective or objective information.

    b. Try to identify all the possible nursing diagnoses that are present in scenario 4. When you identify a nursing diagnosis, also identify an etiology (primary cause) for it as well as defining characteristics.

    c. Use the nursing diagnoses that you wrote in part b and write a goal for each diagnosis that pertains to each domain of learning. When you finish, each diagnosis should have a goal in the psychomotor domain, a goal in the cognitive domain, and a goal in the affective domain.

    d. Write nursing orders and nursing interventions for each goal written in part c. Identify each nursing intervention as dependent, independent, or interdependent.

e. Determine if the goals that you wrote in part c were met completely, partially, or not at all. If the goals were met partially or not at all, determine what could have caused this. (Because this is a fictionalized patient, be creative but realistic.)

NCLEX-Style Review Questions

1. The nursing process will help the RN: (*select all that apply*)
   a. document the ineffectiveness of care implemented
   b. stay organized during data collection regarding the patient
   c. develop a nursing diagnosis to describe the current situation of the patient
   d. implement steps involved in the regimen of nursing care

2. When used appropriately, the nursing process will: (*select all that apply*)
   a. require the use of critical thinking, problem-solving, and use of nursing judgment
   b. maximize errors that can occur during delivery of patient care
   c. ensure the care that is planned and implemented is individualized for the patient
   d. promote the patient's participation in their care by encouraging their autonomy

3. The type of assessment that should occur continuously throughout a patient's health care experience is:
   a. emergency
   b. ongoing
   c. focused
   d. initial

4. The type of assessment that should include only essential data that are relevant to the patient's immediate issue is:
   a. emergency
   b. ongoing
   c. focused
   d. initial

5. The type of assessment that is performed on each symptom as it is identified is:
   a. emergency
   b. ongoing
   c. focused
   d. initial

6. An example of subjective data is:
   a. blood pressure
   b. pulse
   c. nausea
   d. respiration

7. An example of objective data is:
   a. temperature
   b. pain
   c. nausea
   d. dizziness

8. Types of problems that can be experienced by a patient include: (*select all that apply*)
   a. actual
   b. potential
   c. wellness
   d. risk

9. The domain of Bloom's taxonomy that involves feelings, values, and attitudes is:
   a. intellectual
   b. psychomotor
   c. cognitive
   d. affective

10. The domain of Bloom's taxonomy that can be assessed according to distance, time, and speed is:
    a. intellectual
    b. psychomotor
    c. cognitive
    d. affective

11. "The patient will ambulate 6 feet with minimal assistance three times daily." Into which domain of Bloom's taxonomy does this nursing goal fit?
    a. Intellectual
    b. Psychomotor
    c. Cognitive
    d. Affective

12. "Patient will report feeling accepting of her surgical site within two weeks of discharge." Into which domain of Bloom's taxonomy does this nursing goal fit?
    a. Intellectual
    b. Psychomotor
    c. Cognitive
    d. Affective

13. "Patient will verbalize methods of assessing feet daily for signs and symptoms of infection." Into which domain of Bloom's taxonomy does this nursing goal fit?
    a. Intellectual
    b. Psychomotor
    c. Cognitive
    d. Affective

14. The progression of Maslow's Hierarchy of Needs, from lesser to greater, is:
    a. basic physiological needs, esteem needs safety needs, love and belonging needs, selfactualization
    b. basic physiological needs, love and belonging needs, safety needs, esteem needs, selfactualization
    c. basic physiological needs, self-actualization, safety needs, love and belonging needs, esteem needs
    d. basic physiological needs, safety needs, love and belonging needs, esteem needs, selfactualization

15. The RN develops a nursing diagnosis after identifying the patient has a need for self-reliance. This need falls into which section of Maslow's Hierarchy of Needs?
    a. Esteem needs
    b. Love and belonging needs
    c. Safety needs
    d. Basic physiological needs

16. The RN develops a nursing diagnosis after identifying the patient has a need for healthy intimacy. This need falls into which section of Maslow's Hierarchy of Needs?
    a. Esteem needs
    b. Love and belonging needs
    c. Safety needs
    d. Basic physiological needs

17. The RN develops a nursing diagnosis after identifying the patient has a need for self-respect. This need falls into which section of Maslow's Hierarchy of Needs?
    a. Esteem needs
    b. Love and belonging needs
    c. Safety needs
    d. basic physiological needs

18. The RN develops a nursing diagnosis after identifying the patient has a need for adequate nutritional intake. This need falls into which section of Maslow's Hierarchy of Needs?
    a. Esteem needs
    b. Love and belonging needs
    c. Safety needs
    d. Basic physiological needs

19. The RN develops a nursing diagnosis after identifying the patient has a need for freedom from anxiety. This need falls into which section of Maslow's Hierarchy of Needs?
    a. Esteem needs
    b. Love and belonging needs
    c. Safety needs
    d. basic physiological needs

20. The RN develops a nursing diagnosis after identifying the patient has a need for physical safety. This need falls into which section of Maslow's Hierarchy of Needs?
    a. Esteem needs
    b. Love and belonging needs
    c. Safety needs
    d. Basic physiological needs

▶ New Format NCLEX-Type Questions

Ms. Smith arrives for her annual physical examination at the nurse practitioner's office. The nurse practitioner asks the patient to update her on any changes that have occurred in her life over the past year. Ms. Smith's eyes fill with tears as she tells the practitioner that in the past year, she had to retire from her job teaching at a local university to care for her elderly parents. Also, her husband was diagnosed with a degenerative neuromuscular disease that has left him unable to walk without the use of a walker or wheelchair. Ms. Smith tells the practitioner, "It's almost too much for me to handle alone. I have no one to help me."

The practitioner makes a note of caregiver role strain in the patient's chart. The practitioner sets a goal for Ms. Smith as "Caregiver will report an increased feeling of confidence in implementing the caregiver role." The practitioner begins to discuss Ms. Smith's situation with her and discovers that Mr. Smith has a brother living in the same community. "Do you think that he could come over occasionally to help you care for your husband?" asks the nurse. "I never thought about asking him to help; I always felt like this was my job," responds Ms. Smith. The practitioner also writes an order for home health care to assist Ms. Smith with her parents' needs.

The next week Ms. Smith calls the nurse practitioner to tell her that Mr. Smith's brother agreed to come over twice a week to help her with her caregiving duties. Also, she indicates that home health care has already been "so helpful" in working with her elderly parents. "I feel so much better," she tells the nurse practitioner. "I think I can do this now!" The nurse practitioner makes a note of "Caregiver verbalized increased confidence in fulfilling caregiver role."

1. Highlight the section of the scenario above that corresponds to the assessment part of the nursing process. (*hot spot question*)
2. Highlight the section of the scenario above that corresponds to the nursing diagnosis. (*hot spot question*)
3. Highlight the section of the scenario above that corresponds to the planning part of the nursing process. (*hot spot question*)
4. Highlight the section of the scenario above that corresponds to the implementation part of the nursing process. (*hot spot question*)
5. Highlight the section of the scenario above that corresponds to the evaluation part of the nursing process. (*hot spot question*)

▶ Case Study

Review the sample concept map included in Figure 9.3. Add collaborative interventions that could be implemented with the assistance of other departments, such as the Laboratory, Dietary, Chaplain Services, and Discharge Planning, for example. Also, add the nursing diagnoses that you believe to be most applicable.

▶ Concept Map

You are caring for Mrs. Smith, a 58-year-old woman who underwent a mastectomy three days ago. She is scheduled to begin chemotherapy treatments for stage 3 breast cancer in four weeks. She is divorced with one 21-year-old daughter who is in college in another state. When you check Mrs. Smith's incision one morning, you find it to be warm to the touch and reddened at the edges. Mrs. Smith states that the incision seems to be more painful than it was the day before. Create a concept map based on this patient situation.

▶ Note Taker

I. Introduction to the nursing process

A. Assessment

B. Diagnosis

C. Planning

D. Intervention

E. Evaluation

II. Concept mapping

References

Alfaro-Lefevre, R. (2009). *Applying the nursing process: A tool for critical thinking.* Lippincott, Williams, and Wilkins.
Chitty, K., & Black, B. (2011). *Professional nursing: Concepts and challenges* (6th ed.). Elsevier.
Gardner, P. (2002). *Nursing process in action.* Delmar.
Harkreader, H., Hogan, M., & Thobaben, M. (2007). *Fundamentals of nursing: Caring and clinical judgment* (3rd ed.). Elsevier.
Luckowski, A. (2003). Concept mapping as a critical thinking tool for nurse educators. *Journal for Nurses in Staff Development, 19*(5), 225–230.
North American Nursing Diagnosis Association. (2021). *2021–2023 nursing diagnoses.* https://nanda.org/publications-resources/publications/nanda-international-nursing-diagnoses/
North American Nursing Diagnosis Association. (n.d.). *Approved NANDA nursing diagnosis list 2018–2020.* https://ar.israa.edu.ps/uploads/documents/2020/02/4gcM0.pdf
Quan, K. (2007). *The nursing process.* http://www.thenursingsite.com/Articles/the%20nursing%20process.htm
Wilkinson, J. (2011). *Nursing process and critical thinking.* Prentice-Hall.

CHAPTER

10

Spirituality

CHAPTER OBJECTIVES

Upon completion of the chapter, you will be able to:

1. Discuss the process of conducting a spiritual assessment of patients and their family members.
2. Develop the knowledge and practice the skills needed to assess patients' spiritual needs.
3. Identify spiritual nursing care behaviors that could be used in clinical practice.

KEY TERMS

spiritual distress

spirituality

spiritual needs

As the COVID19 pandemic escalated and an increasing number of patients succumbed to the virus, spirituality came into the spotlight as an integral part of holistic nursing care. Burkhardt and Nagai-Jacobson (2016) have described **spirituality** as the essence of being human. Weathers, McCarthy, and Coffey (2016) have indicated that the overall goal of spiritual nursing care is to address the fears and concerns of the patient, alleviate suffering and anxiety, as well as instill hope into the patient. Despite varying definitions of spirituality, experts agree that it is a vital part of forging the caring relationship between the nurse and the patient.

The nurse who intends to ensure that the spiritual needs of each patient are met should bear in mind that spirituality means different things to different people. The **spiritual needs** of the patient and the patient's family include the need to love and the feel loved by others, to feel a sense of belonging, to have a sense of meaning and purpose in life, and to experience a sense of hope, peace, and gratitude. When these needs are not met and the patient is not able to find a source of meaning in life or hope, **spiritual distress** develops instead (Marie Curie, 2019). Spiritual distress can have a negative influence on both physical and mental health.

Conducting a Spiritual Assessment

Kroning and Yezzo (2017) indicated that many nurses feel inadequately prepared to provide spiritual care to patients due to:

- Lack of sufficient interprofessional education
- Work overload

- Inadequate amount of time
- Cultural differences between the nurses and patients
- Ethical issues
- Unwillingness to provide such care

Kroning and Yezzo (2017) conducted a survey of registered nurses regarding the spiritual care provided to patients. Of the nurses who responded to the survey, 90% indicated that they provided spiritual care to their patients, yet only 23% could indicate how that care was provided. This points to the need for nurses to adequately assess their own spiritual beliefs and practices in order that they might sufficiently assess their patients' spiritual needs and therapeutic rituals.

How can a nurse most effectively conduct a spiritual assessment of patients and their families, particularly during traumatic events such as the COVID pandemic? According to the George Washington Institute for Spirituality and Health (2020), the FICA Spiritual History Tool can help with this. This tool consists of an acronym that will prompt the nurse to ask a series of questions, including the following:

- Faith or beliefs
  - What do you view as your primary faith or belief?
  - Do you view yourself as spiritual or religious?
  - What things give meaning to your life?
- Importance and influence
  - Do you view your faith or belief as being important in your life?
  - How does your faith influence how you take care of yourself?
  - How have your beliefs influenced your behavior during an illness (or another crisis)?
  - How will your beliefs help you regain your health (or come through the crisis)?
- Community
  - Do you view yourself as being part of a spiritual community?
  - If so, does the religious community support you spiritually?
  - Is there a person or group of people that you truly love or that you view as being very important to you?
- Address
  - As your health care provider, how would you prefer for me to address these issues as we progress with your health care?

TABLE 10.1. FICA Spiritual History Tool

F	Faith or beliefs
I	Importance and influence
C	Community
A	Address

Developing Knowledge and Skills to Assess Patients' Spiritual Needs

What can individual nurses do to develop the knowledge and skills needed to assess patients' spiritual needs? Hawthorne and Gordon (2019) offer the following suggestions:

- Reflect on your personal beliefs and spiritual views. How are they influencing the nursing care that you provide?
- Practice daily reflection activities that are meaningful to you, such as meditation, prayer, and journaling, for example.
- Participate in spiritually oriented groups with work colleagues. This is particularly important during times of extreme stress such as the COVID19 pandemic.
- Attend continuing programs that pertain to spiritual nursing care topics.
- Promote spiritual care of patients in your facility that extends beyond creating a referral for pastoral care.

TABLE 10.2. How to Develop Knowledge and Skills for Assessment of Patients' Spiritual Needs

1. Reflect on your personal beliefs and spiritual views.
2. Practice daily reflection activities that are meaningful to you.
3. Participate in spiritual-oriented groups with work colleagues.
4. Attend continuing programs that pertain to spiritual nursing care topics.
5. Promote spiritual care of patients beyond creating a referral for pastoral care.

Implementing Spiritual Nursing Care Behaviors in Clinical Practice

Once the nurse has completed a spiritual assessment of the patient and family or support system, how can the nurse implement spiritual nursing care behaviors in clinical practice? Hawthorne and Gordon (2019) noted that initially a trusting relationship must be established between the nurse and the patient. This relationship will set the stage for the additional interventions to be implemented. The nurse should be prepared to demonstrate empathy by attempting to place themselves in the patient's frame of reference. The patient will develop the capacity for self-reflection as the nurse listens to their narrative in a nonjudgmental manner, provides undivided attention, and identifies the patient's strength. As the nurse offers the patient a source of strength and comfort and determines where the patient has received comfort in the past, the patient's hope for either recovery or a peaceful and meaningful death will grow.

TABLE 10.3. Spiritual Nursing Care Behaviors in Clinical Practice

Establishing a trusting relationship between the nurse and patient
Sharing self and demonstrating empathy

Offering hope
Supporting religious practices and beliefs
Referring for pastoral care
Listening with undivided attention and identifying strengths
Being nonjudgmental
Promoting self-reflection

Source: Hawthorne, D. M., & Gordon, S. C. (2019). The invisibility of spiritual nursing care in clinical practice. Journal of Holistic Nursing, 38(1), *147–155. https://doi.org/10.1177/0898010119889704*

Summary of Key Points in Chapter

The chapter discussed the necessity of providing spiritual care to patients and families or support systems. The factors that may cause nurses to feel ill prepared to provide spiritual care to patients were discussed, as was the FICA Spiritual History Tool, which may assist nurses with this assessment. Strategies to assist nurses in developing the knowledge and skills needed to accurately complete spiritual assessments were delineated, as were behaviors to implement spiritual nursing care in the clinical setting.

Conclusion

Spirituality is an integral part of holistic patient care. The nurse leader who wants to model expected behaviors for employees will need to initially develop honed communication skills that will form the basis for the spiritual nursing care to be provided. Communication in nursing will be discussed in the subsequent chapter.

Critical Thinking Questions

1. What do you do in your current nursing practice to practice spiritual nursing care to patients and families or their support systems?

2. Think about a time in your hands-on nursing practice when the situation called for spiritual nursing care to be provided but it was not given. What do you view as the barriers that prevented this? What would you change about the situation to allow spiritual nursing care to be adequately provided?

3. Reflect on your personal beliefs and spiritual views. How do they influence the nursing care that you provide or have provided?

4. Which daily reflection activities do you practice that are meaningful to you?

▶ Scenarios

1. You are caring for Mrs. Smith, a 60-year-old female who lives with her 62-year-old husband. The Smiths have a 32-year-old daughter who lives in another state. Mrs. Smith was recently diagnosed with colon cancer. The tumor was surgically removed today, and she is expected to make a complete recovery. Because of COVIDrelated

restrictions, no one can stay in the room with Mrs. Smith. Use the FICA Spiritual History Tool to conduct a spiritual assessment on Mrs. Smith.

2. You are caring for Joe, a 17-year-old who was injured in a motorcycle accident. His right leg was severely injured and may require amputation. Because of COVID-related restrictions, no one can stay in the room with Joe. However, you notice his parents sitting by themselves in the hospital lobby. Use the FICA Spiritual History Tool to conduct spiritual assessment on Joe and his parents.

▶ NCLEX-Style Review Questions

1. Ways to implement spiritual nursing care in clinical practice include: (*select all that apply*)
   a. offering hope
   b. promoting self-reflection
   c. judging the patient's stage in the grieving process
   d. supporting the patient's religious beliefs

2. You are assessing your patient's spiritual history. You ask him, "Do you view your faith or belief as being important in your life?" The stage of the FICA Spiritual History Tool that corresponds to this question is:
   a. F: Faith or beliefs
   b. I: Importance and influence
   c. C: Community
   d. A: Address

3. You are assessing your patient's spiritual history. You ask him, "What things give meaning to your life?" The stage of the FICA Spiritual History Tool that corresponds to this question is:
   a. F: Faith or beliefs
   b. I: Importance and influence
   c. C: Community
   d. A: Address

4. You are assessing your patient's spiritual history. You ask him, "How will your beliefs help you regain your health?" The stage of the FICA Spiritual History Tool that corresponds to this question is:
   a. F: Faith or beliefs
   b. I: Importance and influence
   c. C: Community
   d. A: Address

5. You are assessing your patient's spiritual history. You are utilizing the FICA Spiritual History Tool and are in the Community stage. A question that corresponds to this stage is:
   a. Do you view yourself as spiritual or religious?
   b. What things give meaning to your life?
   c. Is there a person or group of people whom you truly love or whom you view as being very important to you?
   d. How have your beliefs influenced your behavior during an illness?

▶ Case Study

You are working on the postpartum floor on the 7 p.m.–7 a.m. shift. On your round, you pass by Mrs. Garcia's room and hear her weeping. Your friend Audrey is Mrs. Garcia's nurse. You find Audrey and ask her about Mrs. Garcia. She takes you in the break room and tells you, "I don't know what to do to help her! She delivered a stillborn baby last night and is still here because she had some complications related to the delivery. I've given her some medication to help her sleep and also her antidepressant, but they don't seem to help her. I'd sit and try to talk with her, but I really don't know what to say." What can you do to help Audrey provide spiritual nursing care to Mrs. Garcia?

1. Audrey may feel inadequate to help Mrs. Johnson because of ________. (*select all that apply*)
   a. ____Lack of sufficient interprofessional education
   b. ____Work overload
   c. ____Inadequate amount of time
   d. ____Cultural differences between the nurses and patients
   e. ____Ethical issues
   f. ____Unwillingness to provide spiritual care

2. Audrey wants to develop more knowledge and skills regarding assessment of patients' spiritual needs. What can she do to develop this most effectively? (*select all that apply*)
   a. ____Reflect on her personal beliefs and spiritual views.
   b. ____Practice meditation or prayer.
   c. ____Refer all patients with spiritual needs to the hospital chaplain.
   d. ____Participate in spiritual-oriented groups with work colleagues.
   e. ____Attend continuing programs that pertain to spiritual nursing care topics.
   f. ____Practice daily reflection through journaling.

3. Audrey wants to implement spiritual nursing care behaviors in clinical practice. What should she implement initially?
   a. ____Support religious practices and beliefs
   b. ____Share self and demonstrating empathy
   c. ____Offer hope
   d. ____Establish a trusting relationship between nurse and patient
   e. ____Refer for pastoral care
   f. ____Listen with undivided attention and identifying strengths
   g. ____Be nonjudgmental
   h. ____Promote self-reflection

▶ Concept Map

Create a concept map based on Mrs. Johnson's current situation.

▶ Note Taker

I. Introduction to spirituality

A. Spiritual needs of patients and families

B. Spiritual distress

II. Barriers preventing provision of adequate spiritual nursing care

III. FICA Spiritual History Tool

A. F: Faith or beliefs

B. I: Importance and influence

C. C: Community

D. A: Address

IV. How to develop knowledge and skills needed to assess patients' spiritual need

V. Spiritual nursing care behaviors in clinical practice

References

Burkhardt, M. A., & Nagai-Jacobson, M. G. (2016). Spirituality and health. In B. M. Dossey & L. Keegan (Eds.), *Holistic nursing: A handbook for practice* (6th ed., pp. 135–162). Jones and Bartlett.

George Washington Institute for Spiritual Health. (2020). *The FICA spiritual history tool: A guide for spiritual assessment in clinical settings.* https://gwish.smhs.gwu.edu/sites/g/files/zaskib1011/files/2022-06/FICA-Tool-PDF-ADA.pdf

Hawthorne, D. M., & Gordon, S. C. (2019). The invisibility of spiritual nursing care in clinical practice. *Journal of Holistic Nursing, 38*(1), 147–155. https://doi.org/10.1177/0898010119889704

Kroning, M., & Yezzo, P. (2017, June). Building a bridge to spiritual care. *Nursing Management, 48*(6), 32–39. doi:10.1097/01.NUMA.0000516488.58802.9d

Marie Curie. (2019). *Providing spiritual care.* Marie Curie. https://www.mariecurie.org.uk/professionals/palliative-care-knowledge-zone/individual-needs/spirituality-end-life

Weathers, E., McCarthy, G., & Coffey, A. (2016). Concept analysis of spirituality: An evolutionary approach. *Nursing Forum, 51*(2), 79–96. doi:10.1111/nuf.12128

PART III

Nursing Leadership and Management

CHAPTER

11

Communication as a Registered Nurse

CHAPTER OBJECTIVES

Upon completion of the chapter, you will be able to:

1. Describe the various elements involved in the process of communication
2. Diagram a model of the communication process
3. Discuss the various modes and channels of communication that can be used
4. Describe various techniques found to be particularly effective and ineffective in communicating verbally with patients
5. Discuss strategies for communicating effectively with subordinates, physicians, peers, and upper-level management

KEY TERMS

active listening
channel of communication
communication
decoding
diagonal communication
downward communication
encoding
external climate
grapevine
horizontal communication
incongruent message
I-SBAR-R technique
internal climate
listening
message
mode of communication
nontransactional conversation
nonverbal communication
receiver
sender
upward communication
verbal communication

Introduction to the Communication Process

The process of communication affects every aspect of nursing. Failure to communicate adequately can result in patient injuries, fatalities, and litigation. Marquis and Huston (2012) referred to communication as the most critical leadership skill for the registered nurse (RN) who is moving into the nurse leader or nurse manager role. An RN is required to communicate with a wide variety of individuals daily, including patients, nurse colleagues, superiors such as the nursing supervisor, and subordinates such as nursing assistants. In the 21st century, which came with the advent of email, cellphones, and sophisticated computer technology, this communication is more complex. A statement that may seem straightforward when spoken aloud may be completely misconstrued when written as an email. The ability to communicate both clearly and effectively is a prerequisite to the RN moving forward into a leadership role as the next rung on the career ladder (Marquis & Huston, 2012).

Process of Communication

Marquis and Huston (2012) refer to *communication* as an exchange of information that can occur through speech, writing, signals, or behavior. This exchange of information may mean completely different things for the sender of the message and the receiver, and the verbal and nonverbal messages may seem to be completely disconnected.

Although communication is a complex, multilayered process, certain elements are necessary in order for it to occur:

- Sender
- Receiver
- Message
- Mode of communicating the message
- Encoding the message
- Decoding the message
- Internal climate of the sender
- External climate of the sender
- Internal climate of the receiver
- External climate of the receiver

For communication to occur there must be at least one sender, one receiver, and one message as well as a mode of communicating the message, such as nonverbal, verbal, telephone, or written (Figure 11.1). Encoding occurs if the sender translates their ideas into actual language. Decoding occurs as the receiver interprets the message in an attempt to make it meaningful (Finkelman, 2015). The internal climate exists for both the sender and the receiver and consists of the person's values, feelings, personality or temperament and the stress levels under which the message is sent. The external climate also exists for both the sender and the receiver and consists of the weather conditions, temperature, timing, and overall organizational climate of the facility in addition to the status of the person involved, their level of power, and the degree of authority wielded. Both sender and receiver must be aware of the internal and external climates of the communication process because the perception of the message can change drastically if the climate(s) under which the message is sent changes by the time the message is received. Ultimately, for communication to occur effectively, the sender must verify and confirm what the sender saw and heard as their version of the received message (Marquis & Huston, 2012).

SENDER	MESSAGE	RECEIVER
(internal climate/external climate	(written, nonverbal, verbal)	(internal climate/external climate)

FIGURE 11.1. Model of the Communication Process

Modes and Channels of Communication

For a message to be sent a mode of communication must be used (Figure 11.1). As the sender of the message, the RN will need to select the mode based on the circumstances surrounding the message. As the receiver of the message, the RN will interpret the meaning of the message based partially on the mode of communication used. For example, the written mode has the advantage of literally documenting the exact wording of the message. However, it usually requires more time and considerable skill on the part of the nurse. The RN must have polished writing skills to use this mode of communication clearly to avoid being misinterpreted (Marquis & Huston, 2012).

In comparison, the verbal mode of communication can occur more rapidly but does not allow for the documentation that occurs with the written mode. Also, the verbal mode can allow for subtle nuances of speech and voice intonation not possible with other modes. A variation on this mode is telephone communication, but because the receiver cannot observe the sender's facial expression or body language, the message may be more difficult to interpret. This mode of communication is very dependent on environmental conditions and the mechanical structure of the telephone wiring in order for an intact message to be sent (Marquis & Huston, 2012).

In addition, communication can be nonverbal. This is considered to be the most complex mode in many ways because it includes facial expressions, body movements, and gestures and also communicates the sender's emotional state. As a potential nurse leader, the RN should try to make nonverbal communication consistent with verbal communication; otherwise, the message can be easily misinterpreted (Marquis & Huston, 2012).

Just as a mode of communication is selected for a message, the RN will choose a channel of communication for it as well (see Table 11.1). The channel of communication is the direction in which the message is routed to receivers. For example, when the channel selected is upward communication, the RN sends the message to a receiver at a higher level, such as the nursing supervisor. If the channel selected is downward communication, the RN sends the message to subordinates, such as when a nurse manager discusses a situation with the staff nurses. The channel of horizontal communication is selected when the RN sends a message to others in the organization on the same level as themselves. This is used when a nurse manager discusses an issue with other nurse managers from other units in the hospital (Marquis & Huston, 2012).

A variation of this is diagonal communication, which occurs when the RN interacts with members of other departments in the facility. This could occur when the director of nursing discusses the stocking of a particular medication with the pharmacy manager. Although the pharmacy manager would not necessarily be at a higher level than or have authority over the director of nursing, each recognizes the other as being vital to the functioning of the organization. Finally, the grapevine is considered to be the most informal channel of communication. It moves rapidly and may involve several people simultaneously with no discernible systematic route. The message tends to be distorted as it moves throughout the organization's informal network. Because of the tendency for information to be reported erroneously when the grapevine channel is used, the RN who is a nurse leader must continuously stay abreast of the messages that are moving along this bumpy "information highway" and the personnel who contribute to it (Marquis & Huston, 2012).

TABLE 11.1. Comparison of Channels of Communication

CHANNEL	DESCRIPTION	EXAMPLE
Upward	Message is sent to a higher level	Nurse manager sends message to the nursing supervisor
Downward	Message is sent to subordinates	Nurse manager discusses a situation with staff nurses
Horizontal	Interaction occurs with others at the same level	Nurse manager interacts with other nurse managers in the organization
Diagonal	Interaction occurs with members of other departments	Nurse manager interacts with other department managers in the organization
Grapevine	Informal, message tends to be distorted, may involve several people simultaneously	Hospital's informal information network through which employees may hear erroneous information

Verbal Communication in Nursing

Effective communication in nursing, in its verbal form, is especially important because of its influence on the development of an accurate diagnosis of the patient and the selection of appropriate treatment regimen and its significance to patients, as stated on satisfaction surveys. Elliott and Wright (1999) interviewed former patients who had been seriously ill and found that these individuals described that they heard, comprehended, and responded emotionally to verbal communication even when health professionals assumed they could not understand the communication. These patients reported that they found comfort in having caring words addressed to them, particularly when the sender was attempting to communicate with them as one individual to another.

Macdonald (2001) identified several factors that spotlight the importance of communication by nurses, particularly verbal communication, such as the following:

- Accurate interviewing skills by nurses can produce accurate problem identification.
- Effective communication allows the patient to be cared for as an individual rather than as a collection of symptoms.
- When communication occurs effectively and accurate information is given to patients, research has shown that compliance with drug and treatment regimens tends to increase and patients tend to experience a decrease in stress, pain, and anxiety levels.

The importance of effective interviewing skills on the part of nurses cannot be emphasized enough. When the RN uses a more conversational and exploratory approach to interviewing the patient, the interaction becomes more client-focused and less controlling than the traditional closed-ended, question-and-answer format. An exploratory approach allows the patient the freedom to expand the topics being discussed or even change to a different one entirely. Such interviewing becomes particularly effective when the RN summarizes the patient's verbalized thoughts and feelings periodically, thus demonstrating understanding on the part of the RN, keen interest in the patient's priorities, and a desire to actively discuss these topics with him or her. Various verbal techniques such as the following have been found to be particularly effective when RNs communicate with patients:

- Use open directive questions, such as "How are you coping with the effects of the medication?"
- Use both focusing and clarification simultaneously, such as "You said you have had a great deal of anxiety lately. Please tell me more about the issues with which you are particularly concerned."
- Use empathy and summarizing simultaneously, such as "I sense you are concerned about more issues than only your son's surgery."

Conversely, specific verbal techniques such as the following have been found to be especially ineffective in working with patients because they tend to inhibit complete disclosure:

- Use of leading questions, such as "You're feeling better after that pain medication, aren't you?"
- Use of closed-ended questions that only require the patient to answer yes or no, such as "Are you ready to sit up for a while?"
- Use of advice and reassurance, such as "I'm sure the diagnosis won't be cancer"

Table 11.2 summarizes effective and ineffective communication techniques.

TABLE 11.2. Effective and Ineffective Verbal Communication Techniques

TECHNIQUE	EFFECTIVE/INEFFECTIVE	EXAMPLE
Open directive question	Effective	"How are you coping with the effects of the medication?"
Simultaneous focusing and clarification	Effective	"You said that you have had a great deal of anxiety lately. Are there certain issues that you have been particularly concerned about?"
Simultaneous empathy and summarizing	Effective	"I sense that you are concerned about more issues than only your son's surgery."
Leading questions	Ineffective	"You're feeling better after that pain medication, aren't you?"
Advice/reassurance	Ineffective	"I'm sure that the diagnosis won't be cancer."

Nonverbal Communication in Nursing

Nonverbal communication that occurs between the RN and the patient can be particularly effective and therapeutic. O'Baugh et al. (2009) found that nurses caring for cancer patients who were undergoing chemotherapy treatments frequently used eye contact, therapeutic touching, body movements, and facial expressions while interacting with patients. Smiling was used frequently during the interaction along with humor in an attempt to relax patients during the chemotherapy procedure. The use of therapeutic touch by nurses is particularly significant because it has been shown to decrease stress levels, anxiety, and fatigue in patients undergoing particularly grueling procedures and treatments such as chemotherapy (O'Baugh et al., 2009). In addition, nurses can use observation of nonverbal behavioral cues and facial expressions such as grimacing, clenching and wringing hands, and systematic eye blinking by the patient to know when the individual requires additional pain medication (Shipley, 2010).

A poorly understood aspect of nonverbal communication is **listening**. Consisting of multiple aspects, including empathy, silence, paying attention to the sender's verbal and nonverbal messages, and tolerance and acceptance, it may well be among the oldest skills related to caregiving. Empathy involves being aware of and sensitive to the feelings, thoughts, and experiences of another person—in this case, the patient. Empathy is needed to help the nurse perceive the patient's experiences (Shipley, 2010).

Silence can be frightening for the task-oriented health professional who wants to take action to solve the patient's problem. However, the importance of silence should not be underestimated because its use gives the patient the time and the permission to communicate as needed without fear of being interrupted with unwanted advice and hollow reassurances. The ability to pay attention to both verbal and nonverbal communication as part of the overall listening experience means the nurse is attentive to both the verbal and nonverbal messages sent by the patient and recognizes when they are incongruent (Shipley, 2010).

Paying attention to tone of voice and body language can increase the nurse's degree of empathy, because both help convey the perception of the patient. All previously discussed aspects of listening include the nurse's ability to be nonjudgmental and accepting. This is necessary for the patient to experience a safe environment in which he or she feels secure enough to communicate thoughts and feelings that have gone unexpressed (Shipley, 2010).

The patient is a multifaceted individual who may have a completely different system of cultural beliefs or a lifestyle that is foreign to the nurse. Listening in a nonjudgmental manner allows the nurse to acknowledge this while simultaneously conveying to the patient that there is no need to fear rejection simply because this difference is present. The nurse must actively choose to lay aside all previously held prejudices and preconceived ideas about the belief system of the patient. Without well-honed listening skills, the nurse cannot use reflection and summarization or provide feedback to the patient to convey the message was communicated and understood (Shipley, 2010).

Email

Whereas once written communication in nursing primarily occurred through documentation in a patient's chart, now it can also occur in the form of email. Such a form of communication carries with it its own policies and procedures unique to the health care facility as well as various regulations, not the least of which is HIPAA (the Health Insurance Portability and Accountability Act of 1996), tied to confidentiality and legal issues. Patient names and other types of identifying information should not be used, and diligence should be maintained in guarding passwords, particularly on the part of licensed individuals such as the registered nurse (RN), who could be subject to discipline by the state board of nursing for violation of patient confidentiality.

Email can be used effectively to document a verbal conversation that was held earlier to verify points, clarify any inconsistencies, and summarize the primary result of the conversation. As with any form of communication, it is imperative to observe the socially acceptable guidelines for using it—or, in this case, the "netiquette" that is appropriate. Such netiquette rules are as follows (Finkelman, 2015):

- Indicate if a message is urgent or high-priority and also request a return receipt.
- Specify a subject in the subject line; otherwise, the receiver may assume it is irrelevant.
- Ask before attaching sensitive documents such as contracts to an email; the receiver may prefer to have a hard copy mailed to them.
- Do not use abbreviations, symbols, and emojis in business emails because they tend to make such a communication seem less important.
- Begin the email by putting the most important information first; bullets or numbering may be used to highlight the highest-priority points.
- Be cautious when using color in an email message because some colors may not show up well on a screen.
- When opting to forward a message to another user, include only the most relevant information. Consider if the original sender intended the message to be seen by communicators other than the original receiver.
- When replying to a message, verify that a return communication should be sent only to one recipient rather than as a group reply.
- Verify that messages are received by either requesting a delivery and/or read receipt.
- If an attachment is sent along with a message, verify that the correct attachment is included before sending the message.
- Do not capitalize every word of a message, because this equates to shouting at the recipient.
- Check spelling and grammar before sending any email communication.

Incongruent Communication

Communications that involve both verbal and nonverbal content and use multiple modes and/or channels during the process of sending the message have the potential to be incongruent. An **incongruent message** is one in which the verbal communication does not seem to match the nonverbal message. What should the RN do when incongruent messages seem to be sent? When the patient clearly is communicating one message verbally and a different message nonverbally, the nurse must be on the alert for signals that the patient is ready to provide additional information to clarify the confusing message. The nurse can then make themselves available for the patient to talk more openly. For example, the following conversation between a nurse and a patient contains incongruent communication:

RN: (begins changing bed linen) How are you feeling this morning, Mrs. Smith?

Patient: (depressed facial expression) Oh, I think I'm feeling a little better.

RN: Did the pain medication help you rest last night?

Patient: (turning head to look out of the window of her room) I think so. I woke up early this morning, though. I could hear the change of shift when everyone came in around 6 a.m.

RN: I am so sorry you were disturbed! I'll have to caution everyone about being quieter as they pass by your door early in the morning.

Patient: (looks down at her hands as she winds a paper napkin around her fingers; speaking in a barely audible voice) That's all right. I don't want to be a bother to anyone.

RN: (stops changing bed linen and comes to sit down in chair beside patient's bed) Mrs. Smith, I get the feeling that you don't really feel too well today. Can you tell me about your concerns?

Patient: (turns to look at RN with a distressed look on her face) I do have some things that are bothering me, but I'm really OK. You go ahead and do what you need to today.

RN: (makes eye contact with the patient; takes her hand) Mrs. Smith, you are my priority today. I have plenty of time. You go right ahead and tell me what's bothering you, and I'll try my best to help you.

In analyzing the conversation, it becomes clear the patient, although repeatedly reassuring the nurse that she felt better and had no pressing issues, did in fact have some concerns significant enough to disturb her sleep pattern. The nurse avoided giving the patient false reassurance by telling her truthfully that she was a priority and that the nurse would make every effort to help her. Notice the nurse did not give blanket statements that would be interpreted as false reassurances, such as "I'm sure everything will be fine." Such statements are rightfully interpreted by the patient as evidence that the nurse either does not know how to discuss sensitive issues with the patient or does not see such interaction as being a priority.

Barriers to Communication

Several barriers can make the communication process difficult at best and potentially impossible, including the following (Finkelman, 2015; see Table 11.3):

Failing to listen to the other person involved in the communication can result in negative feelings and responses. This problem can be resolved by practicing active listening, in which the hearer recognizes and acknowledges the person sending the message is conveying an important transmission, whether the receiver agrees with it or not.

Practicing selective hearing occurs when the receiver fails to recognize the needs and problems of the sender. This problem can be resolved by practicing active listening and by making a conscious effort to determine the expectations of the other communicators.

Failing to make further inquiries occurs when the receiver does not request additional information or clarification when the information is vague or confusing. This problem can be resolved by using open-ended questions.

Making judgments occurs when the receiver decides for themselves about the overall value of the message. This problem can be resolved with active listening, making the effort to comprehend other individuals' viewpoints, and pausing before responding.

Expressing opinions while simultaneously practicing intimidation effectively prevents any attempt on the part of the other individual communicating from initiating another message. This problem can be resolved by asking for feedback and consciously being direct rather than aggressive.

Overusing reassurance and/or rejection effectively stops communication. This problem can be resolved by maintaining open communication in conjunction with an attitude of respect for the other individual communicating.

Using a defensive approach conveys that the communicator does not recognize the value of another point of view. This problem can be resolved by remaining open to multiple viewpoints that all have value regardless of whether the communicator agrees with them or not.

Making false inferences occurs when the individual communicating decides on a conclusion without having sufficient information to arrive at such a conclusion. This problem can be resolved by waiting to respond until adequate information has been obtained.

Using personal criticism, profanity, and other types of crude language prevents communication by creating an unsafe and uncomfortable environment in which to communicate. It can more easily be prevented than resolved through diligent monitoring of one's vocabulary.

Initiating spatial issues creates an adequate amount of space between the sender and receiver and avoids intrusion into the other's personal space, potentially disturbing that person's comfort level. Such a problem can be prevented more easily than resolved by being mindful of cultural issues related to personal space, the space that is maintained between staff and a particular patient, and both the ability and the appropriateness of maintaining eye contact.

Maintaining secretiveness can be a very destructive practice in terms of communication because of its interference with trust-building and team construction. This can be resolved through the practice of open communication in which multiple channels of communication are used freely.

TABLE 11.3. Barriers to Communication

BARRIER	DESCRIPTION	METHOD OF RESOLUTION
Failing to listen	Failing to listen to the other person involved in the communication can result in negative feelings and responses being generated.	This problem can be resolved by practicing active listening, in which the hearer recognizes and acknowledges that the person sending the message is conveying an important transmission, whether the receiver agrees with it or not.
Practicing selective hearing	This occurs when the hearer fails to recognize the needs and problems of other individuals communicating.	This problem can be resolved by practicing active listening as well as by making a conscious effort to determine the expectations of the other communicators.
Failing to make further inquires	This occurs when the person does not request additional information or clarification when the information that they have available is vague or confusing.	This problem can be resolved by using open-ended questions.

BARRIER	DESCRIPTION	METHOD OF RESOLUTION
Making judgments	This occurs when the receiver decides for themselves concerning the overall value of the message.	This problem can be resolved with active listening, making the effort to comprehend other individuals' viewpoints, and pausing before responding.
Expressing opinions while simultaneously practicing intimidation	This effectively prevents any attempt on the part of the other individual communicating from initiating another message.	This problem can be resolved by asking for feedback and consciously being direct rather than aggressive.
Using a defensive approach	Use of a defensive attitude conveys that the communicator does not recognize the value of another point of view.	This problem can be resolved by remaining open to multiple viewpoints that all have value regardless of whether the communicator agrees with them or not.
Making false inferences	This occurs when the individual communicating decides on a conclusion without having sufficient information to arrive at such a conclusion.	This problem can be resolved by waiting to respond until adequate information has been obtained.
Using personal criticism, profanity, and other types of crude language	This prevents communication by destroying the environment in which the communication is occurring and making the other person communicating uncomfortable.	It can more easily be prevented than resolved through diligent monitoring of one's vocabulary.
Initiating spatial issues	The amount of space between the sender and receiver can create a huge barrier, particularly if one intrudes into the other's personal space and consequently disturbs that person's comfort level.	Such a problem can be prevented more easily than resolved, and this can occur by being mindful of cultural issues related to personal space, space maintained between staff and a particular patient, and the appropriateness of maintaining eye contact.
Maintaining secretiveness	The maintenance of secrecy can be a very destructive practice in terms of communication because of its interference with trust building and team construction.	This can be resolved through the practice of open communication in which multiple channels of communication are used freely.

Active listening consists of being completely focused on the person who is communicating a message. It includes listening without judgment while absorbing the conversation to such an extent that the listener can repeat to the speaker most of what was intended as the meaning.

Yoder-Wise (2011) noted some guidelines that can be used to further the process of active listening, such as the following:

- Do not allow yourself to interrupt the speaker.
- Gain as much information as possible through listening to prevent misinterpreting the speaker's meaning.
- The speaker's first words may not necessarily represent their genuine thoughts and feelings, so you'll need to listen closely to determine the true meaning of the communication.
- As you listen, detach yourself from your own beliefs and views and judgments to understand the perspective of the speaker.
- Recognize that any prejudices you hold will influence you as you listen to the other person.
- Realize that you must first listen to the speaker and understand their perspective before determining if you agree with that perspective. Effective listening cannot occur without having a genuine desire to grasp the speaker's perspective.

Once we understand what active listening is, we must then determine how it can be used. Active listening should be used as follows (Yoder-Wise, 2011):

- To convey interest in what the speaker is saying
- To encourage the speaker to expand further on their verbalized thoughts
- To help the speaker clarify the problem in their own thinking
- To help the speaker hear what he or she has said in the manner in which it sounded to the listener
- To extract key ideas from a long statement or an extended discussion
- To respond to a speaker's feelings more than to their verbalization
- To summarize the speaker's points of agreement and disagreement to form a basis for more discussion
- To express a consensus of how a group feels after hearing the speaker

Communication With Peers

Once there is an understanding of the process of communication as well as the various aspects of verbal and nonverbal communication, the RN can begin to examine how they communicate with peers, subordinates, physicians, and upper-level management. Communication with peers typically occurs using a horizontal flow of information. This directional flow is due to the equality that is present in the interaction, because no particular person has greater power during the communication. Ideally, there is a sense of trust and respect present and cohesiveness that evolves as nurses work together (Zerwekh & Garneau, 2012).

It is critical that peer communication is accurate when the care of the patient is being transferred to another nurse, such as at the end of a shift, when the patient is having a procedure done, or when the patient is being transferred to another unit of the hospital for care. In these cases, it is essential that all aspects of the patient's care be accurately communicated to the nurse accepting care of the patient. The Joint Commission's National Patient Safety Goals now emphasize that a standardized procedure should be used when communicating such vital information to a colleague in such a situation. Referred to as the *I-SBAR-R technique*, the procedure is as follows (Zerwekh & Garneau, 2012):

I = **Identification:** Identify yourself as the nurse and identify the patient using two methods of identification

S = **Situation:** Describe what is going on

B = **Background:** Describe what led to the current situation and the patient's status before this

A = **Assessment:** Describe what you believe to be happening

R = **Response/Request:** Describe what you believe should happen

R = **Readback/Response:** The receiver acknowledges the information that was given and gives a response

The I-SBAR-R technique's importance cannot be overemphasized because it promotes critical-thinking skills by requiring the sender of the communication to assess the patient and design a recommendation before the communication is actually delivered (Zerwekh & Garneau, 2012). It can contribute significantly to a very effective horizontal flow of information during a communication.

Communication With Subordinates

For many RNs who are promoted into a nurse leader role such as the nurse manager, a challenging part of that role can be learning how to communicate effectively with subordinate employees. For effective communication to occur with employees, nurse leaders must be honest with them about whatever situation is the focus at the moment, create an environment of mutual respect, and work toward a gradual development of a strong bond of trust. An easy and often effective way to develop such respect and trust with employees is to informally communicate for a few minutes each day with each person. It may be no more than a brief inquiry regarding the person's elderly parents and their health issues, for example, but such a query will be meaningful to the employee because it signals personalized interest on the part of the nurse leader. This is frequently referred to as nontransactional conversation, meaning that it is not necessarily intended to have a specific purpose. In addition, if the pace of the nursing unit allows it, the nurse leader may find it particularly effective to meet with the administrative staff one layer down, such as the assistant nurse manager, for example, at least weekly to make certain they are kept up to the minute with developing issues (Belzer-Riley, 2007).

It is also important to recognize the good work of employees, counter any criticism that must be leveled with positive comments, and thank employees for their contribution to a project—and, if possible, publicly. It is particularly important to recognize the significance that unspoken signals can have for subordinate employees. For example, calling an employee into your office to discuss a problem with them emphasizes the difference in the power distribution in the relationship and may affect the dynamics of the interaction that ensues. In comparison, going to an employee's office emphasizes the collegiality that is present in the relationship and may lead to a more open and positive exchange of information even if the communication primarily centers around a problem that has developed (Belzer-Riley, 2007).

One of the most important aspects of communicating with subordinate employees is making the commitment to active listening. This can be implemented with employees through use of several strategies, such as the following:

1. Develop a mechanism for formal feedback: This can be something as simple as a suggestion box. If possible, ensure anonymity so that employees will be more open and honest and can approach you with situations that might not be brought to your attention otherwise.
2. Give serious attention to the information provided by employees: Employees recognize if you use their suggestions and information. If suggestions from employees are never used, at some point, the employees will stop providing them, and the nurse leader will find that a previously busy information superhighway has become a one-way street.
3. Reward suggestions that are used or feedback that is particularly useful: Design some type of reward for employees who take the initiative to make suggestions that help the overall functioning of the nursing unit or that allow the provision of more effective, higher-quality patient care.

Just as active listening has been shown to be an invaluable tool in communicating with patients, it is equally effective to the nurse leader who is communicating with subordinate employees (Belzer-Riley, 2007).

Communication With Physicians

For many nurses, communicating with physicians can be the most difficult part of their daily patient care routine. Nadzam (2009) attributed this difficulty to different communication styles, as nurses are trained to communicate in a manner that is both narrative and descriptive, whereas physicians are trained to communicate in an action-oriented manner that requires immediate attention. The following communication barriers between physicians and nurses have been identified (Nadzam, 2009):

- A lack of structure, policies, and procedures related to verbal reports in terms of content, timing, or purpose of the reports
- A lack of a shared mental model for verbal healthcare communication
- A lack of rules for verbal transmission of information, whether face to face or by telephone
- Difference of opinion among health care professionals regarding what type of information should be communicated during a verbal report
- Frequent interruptions and disruptions
- Frequency with which communication occurs

Merely recognizing that such barriers exist is not a solution to ensuring satisfactory communication between physicians and nurses. The Joint Commission now requires all health care organizations to take steps to improve the effectiveness of communication that occurs between all caregivers, including physicians and nurses, as part of its National Patient Safety Goals (The Joint Commission, 2011). These measures include developing a list of unacceptable abbreviations and reporting critical test results within a specified period.

Furthermore, health care organizations are responsible for ensuring that important information regarding a patient's condition is consistently transferred from one caregiver to the next oncoming caregiver. In addition, specific strategies have been noted to help improve the communication that occurs between nurses and physicians (Nadzam, 2009):

- The nurse should address the physician by name.
- The nurse should have patient information and the chart readily available before attempting to contact the physician.
- The nurse should clearly verbalize any concern regarding the patient as well as the reasons leading to such concern; the physician should recognize such verbalized concern as being valid and worthy of consideration.
- The nurse should develop a potential appropriate follow-up plan; the physician should be prepared to consider such a plan.
- The nurse should focus on the patient's problem when communicating with the physician rather than any extenuating circumstances that may exist; the physician should ensure that sufficient orders are given to deal with the problem at hand.
- Both nurses and physicians should be professional in their demeanor without showing evidence of aggression.
- Both nurses and physicians should monitor the problems of the patient until all such problems either have been resolved in a satisfactory manner or the major exacerbation of chronic disease processes has been eliminated.

Consistent implementation of such strategies may lead to an improvement in the communication that occurs between physicians and nurses.

Communicating With Upper-Level Management

Communication with personnel that serve in a supervisory capacity customarily takes on a formal tone. The message you communicate to your supervisor may well be moved upward along the chain of command to a director of nursing or assistant vice president for nursing, then to a vice president for nursing, and, ultimately, to the chief executive officer. Therefore, to ensure accurate communication, make your message straightforward without being blunt and courteous without seeming to hedge on making a request (Marquis & Huston, 2012).

When communicating with upper-level management, it is extremely important to be assertive without becoming aggressive by expressing your concerns directly and honestly without interfering with the rights of another individual. The assertive individual is capable of stating their views using "I" statements while consciously making verbal and nonverbal communication congruent.

Assertive communication does not include rude or insensitive behavior but does include speaking as an informed member of a profession. What should the assertive RN do when forced to communicate with an aggressive person (Marquis & Huston, 2012)?

1. Use reflection: Reflect the speaker's message back to them, focusing on affective aspects of the message. This allows the aggressive speaker to determine if the situation warrants their use of such highly charged speech patterns and/or anger. Let the speaker know that you are hearing the message that they are sending and that you are paying attention. For example, when communicating with a patient's irate family member, the RN could state, "I hear you saying that you are more upset about this than you have ever been before."
2. Repeat an assertive message: This can be very effective when the aggressor persists in a consistent line of thinking or begins to dramatize the situation. For example, the nurse

manager who is interacting with an aggressive vice president for nursing could remark, "I can see that you're very upset about this, and I'd like to discuss this with you, but not here at the nurse's station. Would you prefer to talk in your office or mine?"

3. Restate the message assertively: Rephrase the aggressive communicator's message so that it is delivered in an assertive manner while eliminating the extreme emotions that were previously included. For example, to a physician who becomes aggressive, the nurse manager could say, "I hear you saying that you consider Mr. Doe's care to be your highest priority, and we certainly want him to have a positive outcome from his hospitalization as well."
4. Pose a question: If the nurse manager is communicating with the vice president for nursing, for example, who is implying that a specific employee may warrant being fired, the nurse manager can assertively ask the vice president if complaints have been received regarding the employee's work performance.

Zerwekh and Garneau (2012) provided the following guidelines to be used by the RN communicating with a supervisor:

1. Keep the supervisor informed of pertinent information on a regular basis. Show a sense of responsibility by gathering important information to share with the supervisor.
2. If you detect a problem developing, have specific information ready to give the supervisor with as much documentation gathered as possible; have several possible solutions to the problem already developed and ready for implementation.
3. Avoid assigning blame, exaggerating, or using an excessive amount of drama in word choices.
4. Do not initiate a conversation when angry, and do not respond to one with anger. Explain your thoughts and feelings on a subject assertively but calmly, using "I" statements.
5. Present an idea for a new project to the supervisor in the form of a written proposal that has all necessary information gathered, and then arrange to meet after giving adequate time for the proposal to be read.
6. Accept feedback whether it's positive or negative and learn from it even if you don't agree with it.
7. Follow the chain of command by taking a problem to the supervisor first before going on to the next link in the chain of command. If you try to bypass this step, most likely the person that you approach will ask if you have spoken to your supervisor about the matter and will send you back to speak to the supervisor before you are allowed to move further.

Summary of Key Points in Chapter

The chapter discussed the use of communication by RNs. The various elements involved in the process of communication were described, and their position in a model of the communication process were specified, including sender, receiver, ending, and decoding. The various modes and channels of communication were discussed, including verbal and nonverbal communication and upward, downward, diagonal, and horizontal communication. Techniques found to be particularly effective in communicating verbally with patients were described, as well as techniques that have been found to be particularly ineffective in such situations. Finally, strategies were offered to stimulate effective communication with

- Subordinates
- Physicians
- Nursing peers
- Upper-level management

Conclusion

Here we discussed the various types of communication the RN may be called upon to use at various points in their career path. Without adequate command of communication skills, sufficient understanding of the process by which communication takes place, and the appropriate type of communication to use in various contexts, the RN runs the risk of not only failing to progress in their career but also sabotaging the current rung they hold on the career ladder.

Accurate communication is crucial to the developing nurse leader, particularly when tasks vital to the care of the patient must be delegated. The intricacies of the delegation process are discussed in the next chapter.

Critical Thinking Questions

1. Write down a conversation you recently had with another person and identify how the communication process occurred during the conversation. Identify the sender, the receiver, the internal and external climates of both the sender and receiver (to the extent that you know such information), the message that was sent, and both the mode and channel of communication. Were you able to determine if the message you sent was the same one received? Why or why not?

2. Create a verbal communication between an RN and a patient that uses at least three effective verbal communication techniques.

3. Create a verbal communication between an RN and a patient that requires the nurse to use aspects of listening: empathy, silence, and tolerance and acceptance. How can you as the nurse determine if your listening skills are sufficiently developed as you care for patients?

4. Create a communication between yourself as an RN and another RN in which you use the I-SBARR technique. Describe in detail what is communicated as the technique is used, including the response from the other nurse.

5. A newly promoted nurse manager is having difficulty working with an assistant vice president for nursing who tends to communicate in an aggressive manner. Develop at least three communication strategies that could be used effectively in this situation and give examples of verbal communication that would use each of the strategies.

▶ Scenarios

1. You are the unit manager of a 25-bed medical-surgical floor. It has been brought to your attention that the staff members are very anxious because a rumor has been circulating through the "grapevine" that the hospital is to be sold. This is not correct; in fact, the hospital will be expanded, not sold, and an additional 25 nurses will be hired.

   Analyze this situation. How do you believe this channel of communication came to be used for this particular message? Whom do you believe has been contributing to use of this channel? What do you believe would have been a more appropriate channel of communication for the accurate version of this message? Be prepared to give your rationale for your answer.

2. You are the unit manager of a six-bed pediatric intensive care unit. One of your patients is a 12-year-old girl who received second-degree burns throughout most of her body when the family home burned to the ground during the night. During the fire, the girl's mother was severely burned, and her father was killed. The mother has been transferred to another hospital for specialized treatment for her injuries. The girl seems to be severely depressed and does not interact in any way with staff as they care for her. She has not spoken since her admission to the unit. You arrange a meeting with your staff nurses to discuss techniques to use in communicating with this patient to increase her interaction, both verbal and nonverbal, with the staff. What suggestions do you believe the nurses would have for this patient?

3. You were promoted to the position of nurse manager of a 10-bed cardiac intensive care unit two weeks ago. One of the staff nurses comes to see you approximately three times a week with suggestions for ways to improve the functioning of the unit. Another staff nurse tells you that the previous nurse manager never interacted with the subordinate personnel and disliked suggestions. Describe at least three strategies for communicating with each of these nurses.

4. You are a unit manager on the oncology floor. One of your nurses comes to you in tears because she says she cannot work with Dr. Lange, the primary physician for that particular floor. You talk with the rest of the staff and find out that all of them have difficulty at times communicating with the physicians who work with these patients. What do you believe will be the most effective strategies to use in communicating with Dr. Lange and the other physicians?

5. As the unit manager of a 30-bed medical-surgical floor, you have recently hired several new staff members. One of them is Carrie, a 30-year-old RN with seven years of experience. Her patient skills are excellent, and she has better IV insertion technique than any other nurse on the floor. However, after Carrie has been on staff for six weeks, you receive complaints from the other nurses as well as the physicians regarding her ability to communicate. Carrie becomes very defensive when a question is asked about her patient care. She normally peppers her speech patterns with profanity and various types of crude remarks. The physicians complain that Carrie does not seem to be listening to them as they give her verbal orders while making rounds. Document a conversation that occurs between you and Carrie in which you have to discuss these problems with her as she ends her probationary period.

NCLEX-Style Review Questions

1. The RN analyzes a message's sender to determine the person's values, feelings, personality, and stress level. The nurse is most likely to classify this as the sender's:
   a. internal climate
   b. decoding
   c. external climate
   d. encoding

2. The RN analyzes the way in which the sender of a message translates their ideas into actual language. The nurse is most likely to classify this as the sender's:
   a. internal climate
   b. decoding
   c. external climate
   d. encoding

3. The staff RN who sends a message to the nursing supervisor is most likely using which channel of communication?
   a. Upward
   b. Downward
   c. Horizontal
   d. Diagonal

4. The nurse manager who discusses a problem on the nursing unit with the staff RNs is most likely using which channel of communication?
   a. Upward
   b. Downward
   c. Horizontal
   d. Diagonal

5. The nurse manager who discusses a problem with the director of pharmacy is most likely using which channel of communication?
   a. Upward
   b. Downward
   c. Horizontal
   d. Diagonal

6. When one staff RN discusses a problem with another staff RN on the same unit, the sender of the message is most likely using which channel of communication?
   a. Upward
   b. Downward
   c. Horizontal
   d. Diagonal

7. An example of an open-ended, direct question an RN could ask a patient is:
   a. "How do you feel about your diagnosis?"
   b. "Are you in pain today?"
   c. "Will you need something to help you sleep?"
   d. "Can you rate your discomfort on a 1-to-10 scale?"

8. An example of a leading question a nurse might ask a patient is:
   a. "Do you have anyone at home to help you after surgery?"
   b. "Are you ready to sit up for a while now?"
   c. "You don't want any more of that juice, do you?"
   d. "How would you describe your childhood?"

9. An example of an RN giving false reassurance to a patient is:
   a. "You seem to have a great deal of anxiety related to your surgery."
   b. "How are you coping with the side effects of the chemotherapy?"
   c. "I'm sure that everything will be fine after your surgery."
   d. "Can you show me where you're having discomfort?"

10. Recognizing and acknowledging the sender of a message is conveying an important transmission even if the receiver doesn't agree with it is known as ______________.
   a. making judgments
   b. practicing selective hearing
   c. initiating spatial issues
   d. active listening

11. When the receiver of a message decides for themselves about the overall value of a message, they are ______________.
   a. making judgments
   b. practicing selective hearing
   c. initiating spatial issues
   d. active listening

12. Failing to recognize the needs and problems of other people communicating is known as ______________.
   a. making judgments
   b. practicing selective hearing
   c. initiating spatial issues
   d. active listening

13. The elements of the I-SBAR-R technique include:
   a. identification, situation, background, assessment, response/request, and readback/response
   b. intervention, situation, background, assessment, response/request, and readback/response
   c. identification, situation, background, assessment, response/request, and repeat/response
   d. implementation, scenario, background, assessment, response/request, and readback/response

14. To improve the communication between nurses and physicians: (*select all that apply*)
   a. the nurse should avoid addressing the physician by name to show respect for them
   b. the nurse should have the chart available before the physician is contacted
   c. the nurse should be professional in their demeanor without being aggressive
   d. the nurse should develop a follow-up plan that could be suggested if necessary

15. When communicating with an aggressive person, the most appropriate communication technique the RN should use is:
   a. leading
   b. clarifying
   c. focusing
   d. reflecting

16. Communication barriers that may exist between physicians and nurses include: (*select all that apply*)
    a. lack of rules for transmission of information either face to face or via telephone
    b. difference of opinion regarding what information should be included in report
    c. frequent interruption and disruptions occurring during communication
    d. congruence regarding how often communication should occur

17. What should the assertive RN do when communicating with an aggressive person who begins to overdramatize the situation?
    a. Use reflection when speaking
    b. Repeat an assertive message
    c. Restate message assertively
    d. Pose a question

18. What should the assertive RN do to help an aggressive speaker determine if the situation warrants the use of anger?
    a. Use reflection when speaking
    b. Repeat an assertive message
    c. Restate message assertively
    d. Pose a question

19. What should the assertive RN do to eliminate the extreme emotions included in an aggressive communicator's message?
    a. Use reflection when speaking
    b. Repeat an assertive message
    c. Restate message assertively
    d. Pose a question

20. The RN has a problem that she believes should be addressed by hospital administration. With whom should the RN speak initially to move up the chain of command?
    a. vice president for nursing
    b. chief nursing officer
    c. medical director
    d. nursing supervisor

▶ Case Study

Today you are working on the oncology floor. One of your assigned patients is for Mr. Jones, a 68-year-old male who has been diagnosed with a form of leukemia. He was admitted for testing purposes after his lab work performed in his physician's office yielded suspicious results. He received his first dose of chemotherapy this morning. During the afternoon, he calls to the nurse's station requesting assistance. When you go to his room, you find that he is short of breath, perspiring, and anxious. He complains of experiencing pressure in his chest. You find that his heart rate and blood pressure are both elevated. You need to notify the physician of the patient's condition. Use the I-SBAR-R technique to communicate with the physician. Identify each element of the ISBAR-R process using this scenario.

1. You are utilizing the I-SBAR-R technique to communicate with the physician regarding Mr. Jones' condition. Highlight the section of the scenario above that would correspond to the "S" part of the technique.

2. You are utilizing the I-SBAR-R technique to communicate with the physician regarding Mr. Jones' condition. Highlight the section of the scenario above that would correspond to the "B" part of the technique.

3. You are utilizing the I-SBAR-R technique to communicate with the physician regarding Mr. Jones' condition. Highlight the section of the scenario above that would correspond to the "I" part of the technique.

▶ Concept Map

Create a concept map using Mr. Jones' situation.

▶ Note Taker

I. Process of communication

II. Modes and channels of communication

III. Verbal communication in nursing

IV. Nonverbal communication in nursing

V. Email

VI. Incongruent communication

VII. Barriers to communication

VIII. Communication with others

A. Peers

B. Subordinates

C. Physicians

D. Upper-level management

References

Belzer-Riley, J. (2019). *Communication in nursing* (9th ed.). Mosby.

Elliott, R., & Wright, L. (1999). Verbal communication: What do critical care nurses say to their unconscious or sedated patients? *Journal of Advanced Nursing, 29*, 1412–1420.

Finkelman, A. (2015). *Leadership and management for nurses* (3rd ed.). Pearson.

Macdonald, L. M. (2001). *Nurse talk: Features of effective verbal communication used by expert district nurses.* Master's thesis, Victoria University, Wellington, New Zealand.

Marquis, B. L., & Huston, C. J. (2020). *Leadership roles and management functions in nursing* (10th ed.). Lippincott Williams & Wilkins.

Nadzam, D. (2009). Nurses' role in communication and patient safety. *Journal of Nursing Care Quality, 24*(3), 184–187.

O'Baugh, J., Wilkes, L. M., Sneesby, K., & George, A. (2009). Investigation into the communication that takes place between nurses and patients during chemotherapy. *Journal of Psychosocial Oncology, 27*, 396–414.

Shipley, S. D. (2010). Listening: A concept analysis. *Nursing Forum, 45*(2), 125–134.
The Joint Commission. (2022). *National Patient Safety Goals*. https://www.jointcommission.org/standards/national-patient-safety-goals/
Yoder-Wise, P. (2018). *Leading and managing in nursing* (7th ed.). Elsevier.
Zerwekh, J., & Garneau, A. Z. (2020). *Nursing today: Transition and trends* (10th ed.). Elsevier.

CHAPTER 12

Delegation

KEY TERMS

accountability
assignments
authority
delegation
responsibility
State Nurse Practice Act
supervision

CHAPTER OBJECTIVES

Upon completion of the chapter, you will be able to:

1. Describe the difference between delegation and supervision
2. Discuss barriers to delegation
3. Describe the process for delegating interventions to an unlicensed person
4. Discuss the process of decision-making
5. Discuss the process of problem-solving

Delegation in most workplace settings would relate to the assignment of tasks by the leader of a project team. However, as a nurse, when a task is assigned by the nurse to be performed by someone else, the nurse retains the responsibility for ensuring that the task is completed appropriately. Failure to ensure that a delegated task is carried out appropriately can literally endanger a patient's life. **Supervision** can be utilized if the person who is responsible for carrying out the delegated task requires guidance (Finkelman & Kenner, 2016).

The legal guide for the who delegates a task is the **state nurse practice act**. Recall that the Nurse Practice Act as well as the state board of nursing have been discussed in previous chapters. Each state's board of nursing ensures that safe nursing is provided to citizens. The Nurse Practice Act in each state describes the nursing scope of practice. The nurse who chooses to delegate a task must ensure that standards of practice are met as well as the policies and procedures of the facility. If the nurse fails to use professional judgment and delegates inappropriately, the nurse will retain accountability for the error (Finkelman & Kenner, 2016).

This means that important issues involved in delegation are accountability, responsibility, and authority. **Accountability** pertains to the person who is willing to answer for the task to be completed. ***Responsibility*** refers to the obligation that is involved when a person accepts an assignment. In comparison, **authority** is the right to assign someone to carry out an act.

Barriers to Using Delegation Appropriately

There are specific barriers that may prevent delegation from occurring effectively:

- Hesitation to delegate because of the nurse's inexperience
- Failing to trust others to do the job correctly
- Failing to apply policies and procedures correctly
- Inadequate amount of time for the nurse to weigh the need to delegate
- Inadequate education and training of the person receiving the delegated activity
- Job descriptions that don't clearly state responsibilities and accountability
- Failing to delegate because of fear that it will anger staff members
- Failing to delegate because of disorganization
- Excessive staff turnover; delegation cannot occur due to constant training of new staff
- Poor communication; this can lead to lack of trust and suspicion
- Delegating when the delegator has little patient contact
- Lack of role models to instruct the nurse on proper delegation
- Staff members who fear risk-taking; this may accompany an inexperienced manager
- Excessive concern over details
- Lack of self-confidence
- Fear of criticism
- Poor relationships with staff members (Yoder-Wise, 2015)

Another aspect of delegation is making **assignments**. This involves the distribution of work that each staff member is responsible for carrying out during a specific work period such as a 12-hour shift. The assignment must be based on the skill of the staff member, the nurse's knowledge and judgment, and the legal scope of practice (Yoder-Wise, 2015).

Delegating an Intervention to an Unlicensed Person

An intervention such as emptying urinary catheters, for example, can be delegated by the nurse to an unlicensed staff member such as a nursing assistant. There is a process involved in delegating an intervention to an unlicensed person:

- The registered nurse (RN) assesses the situation, concentrating on patient needs and acuity level as well as the knowledge, skills, and attitudes of the unlicensed personnel.
- The RN determines which patient needs best fit with the abilities of the unlicensed staff members.
- The RN decides to delegate the task and monitor completion or does not delegate the task and opts to educate unlicensed staff member and supervise instead.
- The RN documents any issues that occurred during task performance as well as the patient's response if applicable.
- The RN provides the unlicensed personnel with feedback on the task performance. If needed, the RN reassesses the situation (see step 1) and intervenes with additional education and supervision (Yoder-Wise, 2015).

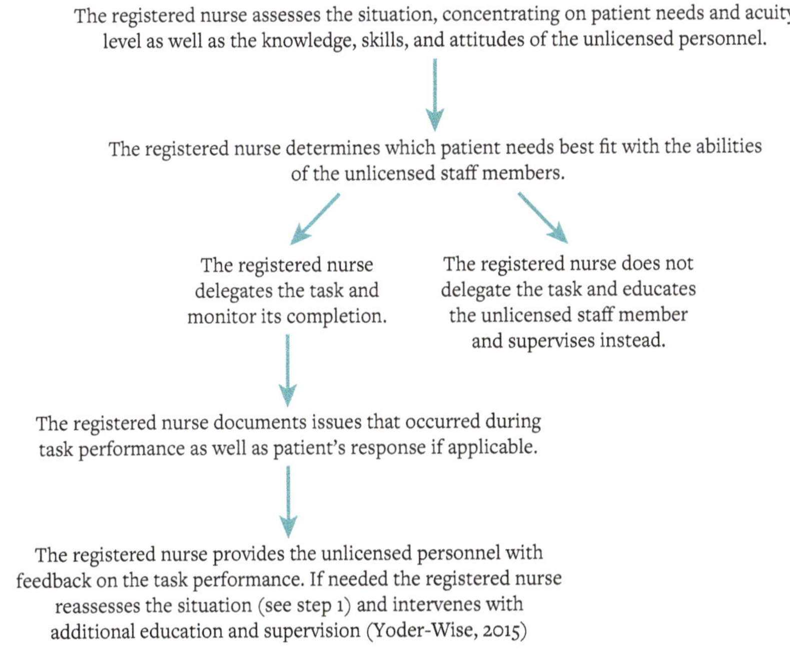

FIGURE 12.1. Process for Delegating Intervention to an Unlicensed Person (Decision Tree)

When the RN considers delegating a task to unlicensed staff members, the nurse must consider:

- Stability of the patient's condition
- Safety of the patient (delegation should not occur if the patient's condition is unstable)
- Degree of critical thinking involved (consider how complex will be the decisions involved to perform the task)
- Time (consider how long the task will take to complete)

Skills Needed to Set Priorities

An important part of delegation is setting priorities. Skills needed to set priorities include decision-making, problem-solving, creativity, and professional judgment.

Decision-making involves:

- Define objectives
- Generate options
- Identify each option's advantages and disadvantages
- Rank the options
- Choose the option that is most likely to achieve the objectives
- Implement the chosen option
- Evaluate the results of the choice made (Finkelman & Kenner, 2016)

Problem-solving involves:

- Define the problem: Decide what is fact and what is interpretation.
- Gather data: Decide what are subjective and objective data.
- Analyze data: Identify possible solutions.
- Develop solutions: Generate as many options as possible.
- Choose a solution: Weight options according to risks and consequences; rank options.
- Implement the solution: Include a contingency plan.
- Evaluate the result: How effective was the planning for resolving this? (Yoder-Wise, 2015)

Summary of Key Points in Chapter

The chapter discussed the process of delegation and its use of accountability, responsibility, and authority. Barriers that could prevent delegation from occurring effectively were delineated. The process of delegating interventions to unlicensed personnel was also described. Finally, the steps in the decision-making process as well as the problem-solving process were discussed.

Conclusion

The multiple facets of the delegation process were discussed in detail. Its relationship to decision-making as well as the problem-solving process mean that conflict may arise at any point. Conflict management is covered in the subsequent chapter.

Critical Thinking Questions

1. Compare and contrast the decision-making and problem-solving processes.

2. What do you view as the three most significant barriers to effective delegation? Explain your answer.

3. How would you go about delegating an intervention to an unlicensed person? Use an example of a situation from your current or previous workplace.

Scenarios

1. Think of a time in your current or previous workplace when delegation did not occur as effectively as it should have. Which barriers to delegation do you see as contributing to the failure of the process?

2. You are considering two different job offers: One is an assignment working 7 a.m–3 p.m. shift on a busy 40bed post-surgical floor in a 450-bed hospital in a large city and the other offer is working 7 p.m.–7 a.m. shift on a small eught-bed cardiac care unit in a 100-bed hospital in the town where you were raised. Use the decision-making process to decide which job offer to accept.

3. You are the nurse manager of a 12-bed Labor and Delivery unit at a 250-bed hospital. The community is experiencing a building surge due to an increase in jobs in an automobile plant.

   You are trying to decide whether you should develop a proposal to increase the number of beds in your unit from 12 to 15 or instead open a small four-bed neonatal intensive care unit. Use the problem-solving process to make a decision.

▸ NCLEX-Style Review Questions

Choose the proper category for each selection.

a. Decision-making
b. Problem-solving

1. ____ Generate options
2. ____ Rank the options
3. ____ Define the problem
4. ____ Implement the chosen option
5. ____ Analyze data
6. ____ Develop solutions
7. ____ Define objectives
8. ____ Gather data
9. ____ Choose a solution
10. ____ Identify advantages and disadvantages

Place the stages of the process to delegate an intervention to an unlicensed person in the correct order:

11. ____ The RN documents any issues that occurred during task performance as well as the patient's response if applicable.
12. ____ The RN assesses the situation, concentrating on patient needs and acuity level as well as the knowledge, skills, and attitudes of the unlicensed personnel.
13. ____ The RN decides to delegate the task and monitor completion or does not delegate the task and opts to educate unlicensed staff member and supervise instead.
14. ____ The RN provides the unlicensed personnel with feedback on the task performance. If needed, the RN reassesses the situation and intervenes with additional education and supervision.
15. ____ The RN determines which patient needs best fit with the abilities of the unlicensed staff members.

▶ Case Study

You are working the 7 a.m.–7 p.m. shift on a busy 40-bed post-surgical floor. You are already assigned to care for five patients, and your nurse manager has just told you that you will be assigned a new patient who is freshly postoperative. Among the staff working on that floor on that day is Sue, a nursing assistant who is still on orientation. You stop Sue and tell her that she needs to assess your patients' vital signs for you because you're running behind schedule in your patient care. About an hour later, your nurse manager pulls you aside to tell you that you were inappropriate in delegating the completion of vital signs to Sue. Where did you err in this delegation? Consider the barriers to successful delegation as well as the problem-solving process to assist you.

1. Highlight the area in the case study that indicates the most significant barrier that is preventing appropriate delegation from occurring.

2. Arrange the steps of the delegation process in the correct order.
   ____ The RN decides to delegate the task and monitor completion or does not delegate the task and opts to educate unlicensed staff member and supervise instead.
   ____ The RN assesses the situation, concentrating on patient needs and acuity level as well as the knowledge, skills, and attitudes of the unlicensed personnel.
   ____ The RN documents any issues that occurred during task performance as well as the patient's response if applicable.
   ____ The RN determines which patient needs best fit with the abilities of the unlicensed staff members.
   ____ The RN provides the unlicensed personnel with feedback on the task performance. If needed the registered nurse reassesses the situation and intervenes with additional education and supervision.

3. Skills needed by the RN to set priorities appropriately include ________________. *(select all that apply)*
   a. decision-making
   b. time management
   c. professional judgment
   d. creativity
   e. problem-solving
   f. leadership

▶ Concept Map

Use the data that you were given in the case study to create a concept map for a standard postoperative patient.

▶ Note Taker

I. Introduction to delegation

    A. Accountability

    B. Responsibility

C. Authority

II. Barriers that may prevent delegation

III. Process for delegating an intervention to an unlicensed person

IV. Factors to consider when delegating an intervention to an unlicensed person

A. Stability of the patient's condition

B. Safety of the patient

C. Degree of critical thinking involved

D. Time

V. Stages of the decision-making process

VI. Stages of the problem-solving process

References

Finkelman, A., & Kenner, C. (2016). *Professional nursing concepts* (3rd ed.). Jones and Bartlett.
Yoder-Wise, P. S. (2015). *Leading and managing in nursing* (6th ed.). Elsevier Mosby.

CHAPTER 13

Conflict Management

KEY TERMS

role conflict
lateral violence
power
bullying

CHAPTER OBJECTIVES

Upon completion of the chapter, you will be able to:

1. Discuss the stages of development into a full-fledged conflict
2. Describe the different types of power
3. Discuss the stages of progression of an existing conflict
4. Describe the various responses to conflict
5. Discuss the difference between lateral violence and bullying behavior

Although conflict cannot be eliminated from the work environment, it can be effectively managed. A common type of conflict in a workplace setting is role conflict. This occurs when there is incompatibility between the expectations attached to multiple roles. It can be very stressful when staff members don't understand each other's roles (Yoder-Wise, 2015).

Stages of Conflict

Conflict ends to occur in four progressive stages:

1. Latent: This is the anticipation of conflict. This occurs when the hospital staff are concerned that there will be a problem with a specific physician because of something that has occurred.
2. Perceived: This occurs as tension begins to develop between people. This is the recognition that conflict is existing at a specific time.
3. Felt: The participants begin to experience anger or anxiety about the conflict. As staff members begin to experience increased stress, they may avoidant behavior to avoid coming in contact with the problematic person. This will prevent the stressful situation from ever being resolved, and therefore the conflict will occur repeatedly, growing only more complicated as additional participants are added.
4. Manifest: The conflict becomes more obvious at this point (Yoder-Wise, 2015).

Types of Power

When staff experience conflict and believe that there is nothing that can be done to change a situation, they may experience powerlessness. Power can be thought of as the ability to influence decisions and subsequently affect behavior (Finkelman & Kenner, 2016).

There are several types of power, such as the following:

- Legitimate: Power is derived from a formal position in an organization. An example would be the power held by the unit nurse manager.
- Reward: Power is derived from the person's ability to reward others when they fulfill certain requirements. An example of such a reward could be a change to a different schedule.
- Coercive: Power is derived from the punishment that is applied when a person doesn't comply as directed.
- Referent: Power is informal and derived from others recognizing a person's special qualities.
- Expert: Power is derived from the person's expertise; the person is capable of providing advice and direction to less experienced staff members.
- Informational: Power is derived from the ability to access and share information.
- Persuasive: Power is derived from the ability to influence others.

TABLE 13.1. Types of Power

TYPE OF POWER	CHARACTERISTICS
Legitimate	Power is derived from a formal position in an organization.
Reward	Power is derived from the person's ability to reward others when they fulfill certain requirements.
Coercive	Power is derived from the punishment that is applied when a person doesn't comply as directed.
Referent	Power is informal and is derived from others recognizing a person's special qualities.
Expert	Power is derived from the person's expertise; the person is capable of providing advice and direction to less experienced staff members.
Informational	Power is derived from the ability to access and share information.
Persuasive	Power is derived from the ability to influence others.

Source: Finkelman, A., & Kenner, C. (2016). Professional nursing concepts (3rd ed.) *Jones & Bartlett.*

A nurse leader will need to have legitimate power and to be able to demonstrate that power. Staff will be empowered by the ability to both participate in and influence decisions.

Responses to Conflict

Conflict is inevitable in a high-stress environment such as that which occurs in health care. There are several typical responses to conflict, including the following:

- Avoidance: This typically occurs when the conflict is with a more powerful person. The person is not able to cope with the anxiety produced by the conflict and opts to withdraw from the situation.
- Accommodation: This occurs when the staff member tries to resolve the conflict by cooperating.
- Competition: The conflict stops because a person with greater power ends the situation.
- Collaboration: All parties involved try to reach an acceptable solution and feel that there's been a positive outcome (Yoder-Wise, 2015).

Once conflict develops, it cannot remain stagnant but will progress. There are typically four stages of progression of the existing conflict (Yoder-Wise, 2015):

1. Frustration: The participants believe that their goals are being prevented from being achieved.
2. Conceptualization: Each participant has a different view of what the conflict is about.
3. Action: This is the response to the conflict.
4. Outcomes: These are the consequences resulting from the actions that have been taken.

Conflict Resolution

How do most people try to resolve conflict? You'll remember seeing these earlier as typical responses to conflict.

- Avoiding: The person chooses not to pursue their own course but doesn't try to help the overall team pursue its goals either. The conflict is postponed.
- Accommodating: The person chooses not to pursue their own course because an attempt is being made to help team members meet their goals. The person who uses this approach tends to develop resentment.
- Competing: The person tries to achieve their own goals at the expense of others. This approach tends to force participants into a no-win situation.
- Compromising: This requires all participants to utilize assertiveness and cooperation. Each person will be able to achieve at least some of their main goals. This includes negotiation.
- Collaborating: This is both assertive and cooperative. Participants work together to find a solution that best satisfies the goals that need to be achieved.

TABLE 13.2. Types of Conflict Resolution

TYPE OF CONFLICT RESOLUTION	CHARACTERISTICS
Avoiding	The person chooses not to pursue their own course but doesn't try to help the overall team pursue its goals either. Conflict is postponed.
Accommodating	The person chooses not to pursue their own course because an attempt is being made to help team members meet their goals. The person who uses this approach tends to develop resentment.
Competing	The person tries to achieve their own goals at the expense of others. This approach tends to force participants into a no-win situation.
Compromising	This requires all participants to utilize assertiveness and cooperation. Each person will be able to achieve at least some of their main goals. This includes negotiation.
Collaborating	This is both assertive and cooperative. Participants work together to find a solution that best satisfies the goals that need to be achieved.

Source: Yoder-Wise, P. S. (2015). Leading and managing in nursing *(6th ed.). Elsevier Mosby.*

We know that characteristics of individuals, interpersonal factors, and organizational factors can all contribute to conflict. A significant source of interpersonal conflict in the workplace is lateral violence. This frequently involves nurses and may consist of verbal confrontations, back-stabbing, undermining, or withholding information. This is not synonymous with bullying since bullying behavior involves an imbalance of power between the instigator and the victim. Lateral violence can be indicative of ineffective leadership, and if it is not prevented from continuing, it can result in a hostile work environment. It is the responsibility of nurse leaders to protect newly licensed nurses from being subjected to bullying behavior as well as lateral violence. This can frequently be accomplished by modeling collaborative as well as cooperative behavior.

How will you know how much conflict resolution has occurred (Yoder-Wise, 2015)?

- How well were the intended goals achieved?
- How realistic were plan that were made?
- How willing were people to work together?

▶ Summary of Key Points in Chapter

The chapter focused on conflict management. Initially the stages of conflict development were discussed as well as sources of power. The responses to conflict were delineated as well as the ways to resolve conflict, both effective and ineffective. The chapter concluded by identifying the characteristics of lateral violence.

▶ Conclusion

Conflict is difficult to avoid completely in a work environment, and particularly in one as highly stressed as that of modern health care. That stress was exacerbated by the pandemic that developed beginning in late 2019. Conflict and subsequent lateral violence may be diminished by appropriate nurse leadership. Supervision will be discussed in the subsequent chapter, and violence in the workplace will also be investigated later in the book.

▶ Critical Thinking Questions

1. You are the assistant nurse manager in an intensive care unit. What do you view as the various types of power that you might exert in this position?

2. One of the staff nurses with whom you work has experienced a conflict with a new physician regarding a patient who has been diagnosed with cancer. The physician is avoiding explaining the condition to the patient and his family members. Which responses to the conflict do you view as being most effective in this case?

3. You work with Sue, a nurse with 10 years of experience in the intensive care unit. Each time that a new employee is hired to work as a nurse in the unit, Sue targets the person with verbal confrontations and backstabbing behavior. As assistant nurse manager, what do you consider to be your best course of action in this case?

4. Compare and contrast lateral violence and bullying behavior.

Scenarios

1. Bill is the nurse manager in the intensive care unit. He has experienced frequent conflicts with Sarah, the nurse manager in the cardiac care unit. You are the director of critical care. Bill has assured you that the conflicts with Sarah have been completely resolved. As his supervisor, how will you be able to recognize that conflict resolution has occurred?

2. Review the situation in scenario 1.

   a. Discuss the different types of power that are being utilized in this situation.

b. Discuss the various responses to conflict that are occurring in this situation.

c. What do you view as your highest-priority actions as the director of critical care?

▶ NCLEX-Style Review Questions

Match the type of power with its characteristics.

1. ____ legitimate
2. ____ reward
3. ____ coercive
4. ____ referent
5. ____ expert
6. ____ informational
7. ____ persuasive

a. Power is derived from the ability to access and share information.
b. Power is derived from the ability to influence others.
c. Power is derived from the punishment that is applied when a person doesn't comply as directed.
d. Power is derived from the person's ability to provide advice and direction to less experienced staff members.
e. Power is derived from a formal position in an organization.
f. Power is derived from the person's ability to reward others when they fulfill certain requirements.
g. Power is informal and is derived from others recognizing a person's special qualities.

Match the type of conflict resolution with its characteristics. Multiple characteristics will match with one type of conflict resolution.

8. ____ avoiding
9. ____ accommodating
10. ____ competing
11. ____ compromising
12. ____ collaborating

a. This is both assertive and cooperative.
b. This requires all participants to utilize assertiveness and cooperation.
c. Participants work together to find a solution that best satisfies the goals to be achieved.
d. Each person will be able to achieve at least some of their main goals.
e. This includes negotiation.
f. The person doesn't pursue their own course or help the team pursue their goals.
g. The conflict is postponed.

▶ Case Study

You are a new nurse on the 7 p.m.–7 a.m. shift on the cardiology floor. You have heard that there is traditionally a high rate of turnover for this area. You have been working on this shift for a month and are considering asking your nurse manager for a transfer to another shift or another area. The team leader for your shift is Beth. Although you successfully fulfilled all of the requirements for a new graduate employee, Beth told your nurse manager that she didn't think you were ready to come off of orientation and needed at least another month of close supervision. She is very critical of all of your activities and insists on watching each procedure that you perform. Last night, you overheard Beth telling the shift supervisor that she didn't think you'd "make it through the first year of being a bedside nurse." Analyze this situation using the information that you have learned about power and conflict management.

1. Highlight everyone mentioned in the case study who would possess the legitimate type of power.
2. Highlight the person who seems to possess the most expert power.
3. Which type of conflict resolution should you try to utilize in this case?
    a. Compromising
    b. Accommodating
    c. Collaborating
    d. Avoiding

▶ Concept Map

Create a concept map based on the situation with Beth.

▶ Note Taker

I. Stages of conflict

II. Types of power

    A. Legitimate

B. Reward

C. Coercive

D. Referent

E. Expert

F. Informational

G. Persuasive

III. Responses to conflict

A. Avoidance

B. Accommodation

C. Competition

D. Compromising

E. Collaboration

IV. Stages of progression of an existing conflict

V. Lateral violence

References

Finkelman, A., & Kenner, C. (2016). *Professional nursing concepts* (3rd ed) Jones & Bartlett.
Yoder-Wise, P. S. (2015). *Leading and managing in nursing* (6th ed.). Elsevier Mosby.

CHAPTER

14

Supervision

KEY TERMS

managerial supervision

personal supervision

Proctor's model of supervision

supervision

CHAPTER OBJECTIVES

Upon completion of the chapter, you will be able to:

1. Discuss factors that characterize effective clinical supervision
2. Describe the effect that effective clinical supervision can make in the workplace
3. Describe barriers to effective clinical supervision
4. Describe ways to eliminate barriers to effective clinical supervision

Supervision

Many nurse leaders began their careers with a position as a clinical nurse supervisor. Most nurses have a clear picture of what ineffective supervision encompasses, but when asked what makes an effective supervisor, they become less certain. **Supervision** in nursing can be thought of as an ongoing professional relationship between at least two staff members with differing levels of expertise. Primary purposes of supervision include, most significantly, that of ensuring patient safety along with the promotion of professional development and the enhancement of knowledge and skills (Rothwell et al., 2021). **Proctor's model of supervision** emphasized three major functions: managerial/administrative, educational, and supportive. All three functions should be occurring simultaneously with flexibility and overlap being obvious (Proctor, 2008).

Rothwell et al. (2021) has suggested several forms of supervision occur: internal managerial, internal reflective, external professional, and external personal. These can be viewed on a continuum with **managerial supervision** occurring within the organization and focusing on task and processes, while **personal supervision** occurs at the worker level and focuses on the worker's narrative that is brought into the situation. Personal supervision is significant because it provides a safe place for workers to connect with others and self-reflect while verbalizing their feelings. It usually allows a more intensive focus on clinical issues and personal professional development rather than on the concerns of the organization. In the case of nursing, when the clinical supervisor is also a line manager such as a charge nurse, there is a focus on learning and development of nurses as well as a simultaneous focus on service delivery, risk management, and underperforming benchmarks.

Developing Effective Clinical Supervision

Which factors promote the development of effective clinical supervision?

- Safe and supportive environment: This promotes the development of mutual trust. It is important for supervisors to have sufficient time to discuss the needs of individual workers. There also needs to be time for practice-related issues to be discussed, particularly those pertaining to ethical concerns.
- Regular supervision with constructive feedback: It was found that workers valued supervision received on a regular basis as well as constructive feedback that gives them the opportunity to reflect on their practice. Supervisors who give real-time feedback as well as confirmation when staff have been especially effective were found to be particularly valuable. Supervisors that are viewed as being experts in their field tend to be seen as having credibility and being worthy of workers' trust.
- Supervisor training: Supervisors need to receive training in cultural competence as well as problemsolving (Rothwell et al., 2021).

How much of a difference can effective clinical supervision make in the workplace?

- Staff retention: Studies have found that effective supervision can result in staff retention, improved job satisfaction, improved staff well-being, as well as an improvement in workers' perception of being valued.
- Reduced stress: Effective supervision can reduce work anxiety since the environment will promote the sharing of skills, knowledge, and resources.
- Improved working environment: Effective supervision can improve the implementation of workplace policies because of improved understanding of the reason for the policies. Supervision with nurse managers has been found to improve communication among staff.
- Increased quality of care delivery: Studies showed that with direct supervision of nurses, there tended to be a great degree of compliance with protocols, and subsequently patient outcomes improved (Rothwell et al., 2021).

Barriers to Effective Clinical Supervision

Once the characteristics and benefits of effective clinical supervision in nursing are known, we must look at the barriers that can prevent such supervision from being utilized. Barriers to effective clinical supervision include:

- Lack of time and increased workload: Supervisors with an extremely busy work environment may find decreased opportunities for the reflection with staff members needed to strengthen developing trust relationships. Staff, particularly new employees and new graduate nurses, may be left struggling to navigate their own way through policies and protocols.

- Inadequate staffing: Key factors that can hinder development of effective clinical supervision have been found to include the location of the facility such as in rural communities where there are fewer staff and also shift work patterns.
- Inadequate support from organizational management: When management do not focus on supervision as an important function in the organization, there will not be sufficient time and resources devoted to developing staff members into potential supervisors.
- Lack of supervisor training: As was previously mentioned, a lack of sufficient resources can lead to inadequate training of supervisors. The end result of such inadequate training can be poor-quality supervision due to supervisors' unfamiliarity with their responsibilities, the policies and protocols of the facility, and any accreditation requirements.
- Lack of support when faced with underperforming staff: A stressed and harassed supervisor may be unaware that a staff member does not possess sufficient knowledge or a skill level needed to fulfill the requirements of a task. Supervisors faced with trying to fill an increasing number of vacant nursing positions, particularly when faced with a crisis such as the recent pandemic, may be hesitant to give negative feedback to employees for fear that the staff member will resign (Rothwell et al. 2021).

What can be done to detect and hopefully eliminate barriers to successful supervision? Sellers et al. (2016) noted that significant issues that tend to occur during the supervisory process include lack of organization and time management, inadequate interpersonal skills, and difficulty accepting constructive criticism.

- The employee who is disorganized tends to miss deadlines and may be late to meetings. The supervisor who is working with the disorganized employee should determine if the employee exhibits poor time management regarding all aspects of their life or only regarding a special project. In the hopes of decreasing the lack of organization and also providing support to the employee, the supervisor can introduce the employee to various online organizational tools such as email and cell phone reminders as well as tips that include using daily to-do lists and color-coding tasks according to importance.
- The employee who demonstrates poor interpersonal skills may demonstrate inappropriate language, arguing, or inadequate eye contact. The supervisor who is working with the employee who lacks interpersonal skills should assess the person carefully to determine the specific skills that are lacking, such as effective speaking, writing, and active listening for example. In an attempt to improve the employee's interpersonal skills and provide support to the employee, the supervisor can provide access to tools such as assertiveness training, a course on business and professional writing, and potentially even role play of difficult client situations.
- The employee who has difficulty accepting constructive criticism may argue frequently with the supervisor or demonstrate overly emotional reactions such as becoming defensive or crying in response to feedback. When attempting to help the employee reaction more appropriately to receiving criticism, the supervisor should initially use self-reflection to determine if the supervisor has been overly harsh in providing feedback. The criticism

delivered should match the employee's behavior in question. If the supervisor knows that significant criticism will be delivered, the supervisor should reassure the employee that the person will have the opportunity to ask questions and respond to all of the supervisor's concerns. If the employee begins to become overly emotional during the evaluative session, the supervisor can offer the person the opportunity to step out of the room for a few moments to compose themselves.

▸ Summary of Key Points in Chapter

The chapter discussed a definition of supervision in nursing, emphasizing Proctor's model of supervision. Factors promoting the development of effective clinical supervision were discussed, along with the effect that such supervision can make in the workplace. Barriers to effective clinical supervision in nursing were delineated along with possible ways to eliminate them.

▸ Conclusion

The nurse supervisor who is striving to become more effective at the overall process of supervision will find that this is a process that extends throughout the career as a nurse leader. The supervisory skills will hopefully become honed as the supervisor encounters new challenges in the workplace. The nurse supervisor will usually also participate in some form of quality improvement in the health care facility where that person is employed. Quality improvement is discussed in detail in the subsequent chapter.

▸ Critical Thinking Questions

1. Compare and contrast the type of supervision provided to the employee who is chronically late with the employee who demonstrates poor interpersonal skills.

2. What type of supervision would you provide for the employee who cannot receive constructive criticism without becoming defensive and weeping?

3. Compare and contrast managerial supervision with personal supervision.

4. Provide examples of constructive and nonconstructive feedback.

5. Consider the barriers to effective supervision. Rank them according to your view of their influence on supervision. Be prepared to defend your selection.

   a. ____ Lack of time and increased workload

   b. ____ Inadequate staffing

   c. ____ Inadequate support from organizational management

   d. ____ Lack of supervisor training

   e. ____ Lack of support when faced with underperforming staff

▶ Scenarios

1. Consider your current or former workplace.
   a. Which characteristics does it possess that would promote effective nursing clinical supervision?
   b. Which of the characteristics does the facility lack most significantly?
   c. Which barriers to development of effective nursing supervision does your facility exhibit?
2. You are a brand-new nursing supervisor. Unfortunately, the facility doesn't have enough staff to spare you to attend supervisor training. What could you do to enhance your ability to supervise effectively?

3. Your facility is severely understaffed. As a nursing supervisor, you are being pressured to avoid giving negative feedback on staff evaluations to prevent nurses from potentially resigning to go to more lucrative positions elsewhere. What could you do to enhance your ability to supervise effectively?

4. Several of the employees that you supervise as a new nurse supervisor are chronically late for each shift that they work. As the supervisor, what could you do to supervise these staff members most effectively and potentially decrease this problem?

5. Several of the employees that you supervise as a new nurse supervisor argue with you any time that you need to talk with them about a critical issue. As the supervisor, what could you do to supervise these staff members most effectively and potentially decrease this problem?

NCLEX-Style Review Questions

1. Which factors promote the development of effective clinical supervision? (*Select all that apply*)
   a. ____ Staff retention
   b. ____ Safe and supportive environment
   c. ____ Regular supervision with constructive feedback
   d. ____ Inadequate support from management
   e. ____ Increased quality of care delivery

2. Match the type of employee with the appropriate supervisory techniques to be utilized.
   a. Employee is disorganized
   b. Employee has poor interpersonal skills
   c. Employee has difficulty accepting constructive criticism

   ____ Use self-reflection
   ____ Color-code tasks
   ____ Assess employee's speaking, writing, and active listening skills
   ____ Utilize to-do lists
   ____ Reassure the employee that there will opportunity for questions
   ____ Provide access to assertiveness training
   ____ Utilize email and cell phone reminders
   ____ Give the employee the opportunity to leave the room to compose themselves
   ____ Provide access to a course on business and professional writing
   ____ Provide role-play of difficult client situations

Case Study

You were recently promoted to nursing supervisor on the 7 p.m.–7 a.m. shift. Your first shift in your new position begins tonight. The administrator has told you that once the facility is better staffed, you will be sent to a three-day seminar on supervisor training. You arrive at 6:30 p.m. to get report from the previous shift supervisor. You are concerned to see how harassed Joe, the 7 a.m.–7 p.m. supervisor, looks. He tells you, "You'd better go talk to Dr. Martin in Nursing Administration first thing. He's got one of the new graduate nurses in there demanding that she be fired because she was a little uncertain when interpreting an EKG strip in front of him. She's crying, and he's screaming! It's a mess." Joe also tells you that the other issue that will be high-priority for the night will be overseeing the staff on 7 West. That floor just underwent a huge staff turnover and has a new nurse manager and shift charge nurse. The shift charge nurse is threatening to resign because the staff won't work with her. They recently received permission to use a self-scheduling staffing model, but now no one will sign up to work the shifts. You sigh and start making another pot of coffee. It's going to be a long night.

1. What do you consider to be your initial priority in this scenario? Be able to support your answer.

2. What are the factors present that would promote effective clinical supervision?

3. What are the barriers that would prevent effective clinical supervision from occurring?

4. Highlight all areas in the case study that are reflective of a barrier to adequate supervision.

▶ Concept Map

Design a concept map that reflects your current situation as a supervisor.

▶ Note Taker

I. Proctor's model of supervision

II. Forms of supervision

III. Factors that promote development of effective clinical supervision

A. Safe and supportive environment

B. Regular supervision with constructive feedback

C. Supervisor training

IV. Effect of effective clinical supervision in the workplace

A. Staff retention

B. Reduced stress

C. Improved working environment

D. Increased quality-of-care delivery

V. Barriers to effective clinical supervision

A. Lack of time and increased workload

B. Inadequate staffing

C. Inadequate support from organizational management

D. Lack of supervisor training

E. Lack of support when faced with underperforming staff

VI. Issues that tend to occur during the supervisory process

A. Lack of organization and time management

B. Inadequate interpersonal skills

C. Difficulty accepting constructive criticism

References

Proctor, B. (2008). *Group supervision: A guide to creative practice.* Sage.

Rothwell, C., Kehoe, A., Farook, S. F., & Illing, J. (2021). Enablers and barriers to effective clinical supervision in the workplace: A rapid evidence review. *BMJ Open, 11*, e052929. doi: 10.1136/bmjopen-2021-052929

Sellers, T. P., LeBlanc, L. A., & Valentino, A. L. (2016). Recommendations for detecting and addressing barriers to successful supervision. *Behavior Analysis in Practice, 9*(4), 309–319. https://doi.org/10.1007/s40617-016-0142-z

CHAPTER

15

Quality Improvement

CHAPTER OBJECTIVES

Upon completion of the chapter, you will be able to:

1. Recognize the current benchmarks being used within a health care organization
2. Discuss how to measure performance according to systems, processes, and outcomes
3. Describe the process of root case analysis
4. Create a fishbone diagram
5. Complete a 5-why analysis

KEY TERMS

benchmark
fishbone diagram
5-why analysis
outcome measure
performance measurement
process measure
root cause analysis
sentinel event

The recent pandemic and the resulting complications in health care have made the need for quality improvement in nursing more evidence than ever before. In recent years, quality monitoring in health care has had various names, including quality assurance, total quality management, quality improvement, continuous quality improvement, and performance improvement. Accrediting entities expect hospitals and other health care facilities to continuously strive to provide the highest possible quality of care. Performance monitoring is based on data collected. When a hospital compares its current performance with its own historical data or with data from similar organizations, it establishes a benchmark or best practice for a specific process. Establishing a benchmark for each performance measure that is monitored allows the hospital to set performance baselines, describe the performance stability, and identify the areas that will need more detailed data collection (Shaw et al., 2012).

Performance Measurement

Performance measurement in health care can show an organization's performance pertaining to a process or outcome. Specifically, performance will be measured in:

- Systems: This includes buildings, equipment, professional staff, and policies.
- Processes: This includes all the interrelated activities in a health care organization that promotes effective patient care outcomes.

- Outcomes: This includes the patient's expectations, needs, and quality of life resulting from care, treatment, and services.

To determine the systems, processes, and outcomes that need to be improved, the health care organization must determine whether the needs and expectations of its customers are being met. Performance measures must be identified. A process measure focuses on delivering services that will lead to a specific outcome. An example of a process measure would be the percentage of deliveries through cesarean section. An outcome measure shows the result of the performance or nonperformance of a function or process. One example of an outcome measure would be the incidence of postoperative wound infections when antibiotics are utilized. Benchmarking can assist in identifying systems, processes, and outcomes for improvement. It consists of comparing the products, services, and outcomes of one organization with those of a similar organization. Benchmarking based on best practice or state or national standards helps the organization determine whether processes fall within the acceptable norm. A hospital can receive information about an ineffective care process through a sentinel event. Sentinel events usually involve significant injury or death of a patient or employee due to a preventable cause (Shaw et al., 2012).

Sentinel Events

A sentinel event can be investigated using a root cause analysis. The root cause analysis is the most basic factor that, if corrected, will prevent reoccurrence of the situation that produced the sentinel event. The process of root cause analysis consists of several steps:

- Clearly define the undesired outcome: It may be necessary to review the organization standard and compare it with the event that occurred to clarify the problem.
- Collect the data: Begin interview immediately while details are still fresh.

Questions to Be Asked to Determine the Details Regarding the Undesired Outcome:

1. When did the event occur?
2. Where did the event occur?
3. What conditions were present before the event occurred?
4. What barriers could have prevented the event from occurring?
5. What are all the potential causes of the event?
6. What actions could prevent a recurrence of the event?

- Create an event and causal factor chart: Causal factors can be human errors or system failures, for example. If eliminated, these factors that could have prevented the event from occurring or at least from being as serious. Charting the causal factors allows investigators to organize the information that has been gathered and to identify any gaps in knowledge. A tool that can be helpful at this stage is the fishbone diagram. It allows investigators to identify factors related to the event. The head of the fishbone is the undesired occurrence and the branches attached to the skeleton are major factors that failed, such as people, equipment, supplies, or processes. This cause-and-effect diagram must consider all possible causes and each one must be reviewed and backed with sufficient data. All of the potential causes must be prioritized according to their contribution to the event.

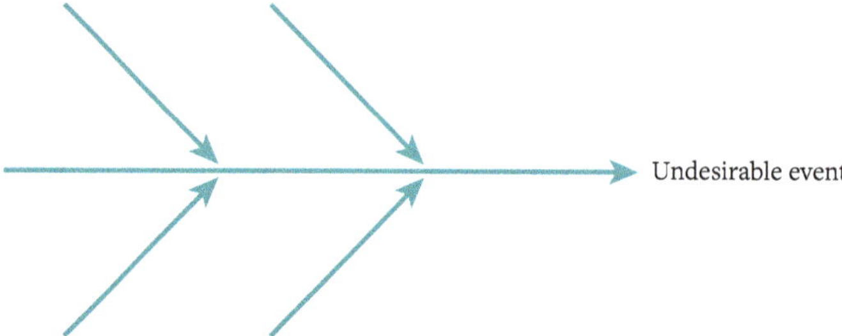

FIGURE 15.1. Fishbone Diagram

When all possible causes have been identified, utilize the 5-why analysis to determine the root cause.

Completing the 5-Why Analysis:

1. Write down a potential cause of the unwanted outcome.
2. Ask why the problem happened and write the answer below the problem.
3. If the root cause was not identified in step 2, ask "Why" again and write that answer below the problem.
4. Continue step 3 until the investigators agree that the root cause of the problem has been identified.
5. Review the data collection that took place during steps 1–4.

The 5-why analysis is discontinued when the root cause is identified, data are inadequate to continue the process, or investigators determine that the problem isn't correctable (Axley d& Robbins, 2009).

- Identify the root cause: This may involve the use of a decision diagram to identify the reasons for each factor. Investigators must ask if the occurrence in question was corrected, was eliminated, or could have been avoided. If the undesired outcome could have been avoided, it will have been considered a root cause and should be kept in the diagram. In some situations, it will be difficult to be completely certain that an event or a condition is a cause because the data needed to provide certainty are not completely accessible. In such a case, the investigators will consider the cause to be "probable" since there is considerably more evidence to consider it as a cause than not. The probable causes should remain as part of the decision diagram until disproved.
- Present recommendations generated from the investigation: Corrective actions should be applied to eliminate proximate causes and mitigate the negative effects of the root causes. The cause-and-effect diagram should be analyzed to help in setting priorities to arrange causes according to importance. Recommendations for corrective actions should include a timeline for implementing changes, monitoring the progress of strategies, and the application of outcome measures (Axley & Robbins, 2009).

Summary of Key Points in Chapter

The chapter discussed performance measurement according to systems, processes, and outcomes. The process of root cause analysis to investigate a sentinel event was reviewed.

In addition, the creation of a fishbone diagram along with completion of a 5-why analysis was described as part of the investigatory process.

Conclusion

There are many other processes and tools that can be utilized in quality improvement, but the success of the overall process depends most on the consistency of the data collection. Regardless of the variety of tools that are utilized, if data are not collected effectively, efficiently, and consistently, the quality of patient care outcomes will suffer, and needed changes in health care delivery will not be made. The various health care delivery systems will be discussed in the subsequent chapter.

Critical Thinking Questions

1. Consider your current or a former workplace. What are some benchmarks that are being utilized in this facility?

    a. Which benchmarks are performing at an expected level? Explain why you consider them to be performing at this level.

    b. Which benchmarks would you consider to be underperforming? Explain why you consider them to be underperforming.

2. How would this facility measure performance according to systems, processes, and outcomes?

3. Describe a sentinel event that occurred in this facility.

4. Discuss the steps of the process of root cause analysis.

5. How would you apply the steps of the root cause analysis process to the sentinel event that you discussed in question 3?

Scenarios

1. You are working as a nurse in Mercy Hospital when a sentinel event occurs: A medication is administered to a patient in error, and the patient has died. The medication was administered by a nurse who was pulled in to assist from another floor.

   a. Work through the steps of the root cause analysis process.

   b. How will you determine the details of the undesired outcome?

   c. Create a fishbone diagram.

   d. Complete the 5-why analysis regarding this situation.

   e. What would you view as some potential corrective actions that could be applied?

2. You are working as a nurse in Mercy Hospital when a sentinel event occurs: A series of errors take place in surgery, and a patient's right leg is removed when, in fact, the left leg should have been removed.

   a. Work through the steps of the root cause analysis process.

   b. How will you determine the details of the undesired outcome?

   c. Create a fishbone diagram.

   d. Complete the 5-why analysis regarding this situation.

   e. What would you view as some potential corrective actions that could be applied?

▶ NCLEX-Style Review Questions

1. Arrange the steps of the root cause analysis process as they should occur.
   ____ Create an event and causal factor chart
   ____ Clearly define the undesired outcome
   ____ Present recommendations generated from the investigation
   ____ Collect the data
   ____ Identify the root cause

2. Establishing a benchmark for each performance measure that is monitored allows the hospital to: (*select all that apply*)
   a. set performance baselines
   b. make effective staffing decisions
   c. describe the performance stability
   d. identify areas requiring detailed data collection

3. Performance that is being measured in systems includes: (*select all that apply*)
   a. patient's expectations
   b. buildings
   c. needs
   d. equipment
   e. professional staff
   f. quality of life resulting from care
   g. policies

4. Performance that is being measured in outcomes includes: (*select all that apply*)
   a. patient's expectations
   b. buildings
   c. needs
   d. equipment
   e. professional staff
   f. quality of life resulting from care
   g. policies

▶ Case Study

You are working as a registered nurse on 5-North, a busy 40-bed medical oncology floor. You completed your Bachelor's in Nursing program six months ago. You are working with Jean, a registered nurse with 20 years of experience as a nurse who has been working in a hospital environment for only about three months. She previously worked in a variety of community health settings. Jean tells you, "Do you remember when Mr. Smith in Room 505 fell on the night shift and nobody found him until hours later? He was an older man, about 82 years old, I think. I heard that he died as a result of the fall and the family is suing the hospital! I also heard that the Quality Management department is doing a root-cause analysis. Do you know how that works? I've never been through one of those in a hospital before."

1. Outline the root cause analysis process for Jean using Mr. Smith's situation.

2. Highlight the section of the scenario that corresponds to the undesired outcome.

3. Highlight the section of the scenario that be included with the data collection.

4. A 5-why analysis is being completed as part of the root cause analysis process. The 5-why analysis will be discontinued when: (*select all that apply*)
   a. ____ data are inadequate to continue the process
   b. ____ investigators determine that the problem isn't correctable
   c. ____ the patient is not cooperative with the process
   d. ____ the root cause is identified

▶ Concept Map

Create a concept map using Mr. Smith's situation pertaining to the fall in the hospital. He was originally admitted to the hospital with a diagnosis of congestive heart failure so that a new medication could be started on him while he was being closely monitored.

▶ Note Taker

I. Benchmarks

II. Performance measurement

A. System

B. Process

C. Outcome

III. Root cause analysis

A. Define undesired outcome

B. Collect data

C. Create an event and causal factor chart

1. Fishbone diagram

2. 5-why analysis

D. Identify the root cause

E. Present recommendations generated from the investigation

References

Axley, B., & Robbins, K. (2009). *Applying continuous quality improvement in clinical practice.* American Nephrology Nurses Association.

Shaw, P., Elliott, C., Isaacson, P., & Murphy, E. (2012). *Quality and performance improvement in healthcare: A tool for programmed learning.* American Health Information Management Association.

CHAPTER

16

Health Care Delivery Systems

CHAPTER OBJECTIVES

Upon completion of the chapter, you will be able to:

1. Discuss the various types of managed care organizations
2. Describe the advantages of an integrated delivery system
3. Discuss the benefits of implementing telehealth
4. Discuss the effect of the pandemic on telehealth

KEY TERMS

deductible
exclusive provider organization plan
health maintenance organization
integrated delivery system
managed care organizations
point-of-service plan
preferred provider organization
preferred providers
self-directed services
telehealth

The current health care delivery system in the United States consists of health practitioners, agencies, and organizations, all of which share the goal of delivering health care yet operate on an independent basis. Most patient services are provided by physicians who sell services on a fee-for-service basis. Many Americans have health insurance benefits through their employers. These benefits are a result of contributions from both the employee and the employer. As the number of citizens without health insurance increases yearly, the cost of providing health care also increases (Cockerham, 2008).

Managed Care Organizations

Managed care organizations are entities that strive to reduce health care expenditures costs. Versions of managed care organizations include the exclusive provider organization plan, preferred provider organization, health maintenance organization, and point-of-service organizations (Heaton & Tadi, 2021).

An exclusive provider organization plan (EPO) is a type of health insurance plan that requires members to utilize specific health care providers except when an emergency exists. Such plan typically only covers services that are provided by providers that are within the network. Remaining within the network can result in lowered costs to the consumer. Health insurers negotiate the payment terms with health care providers and facilities to create a network of providers that participate in the plan. Usually consumers are not required to choose a primary care physician or obtain referrals to see specialists. Prior authorization may be required for the EPO to cover some services such as hospitalization and specific medications (Gordon, 2021).

In addition, a **preferred provider organization (PPO)** is a health insurance plan that involves networks composed of health insurance companies as well as contract medical professionals. Health care facilities and practitioners that are known as ***preferred providers*** will provide services to the plan's policyholders at a reduced rate. Plan subscribers receive the maximum benefit when they visit health care professionals who are within the network; they can also receive coverage when utilizing out-of-network providers. PPO plans tend to charge higher premiums because they cost more to administer and manage. Participants usually are charged a copayment, which is paid to the health care provider upon each visit. The plan participant will also be required to meet a **deductible** before the plan begins paying claims in entirety. Patients will be allowed to visit out-of-network facilities at a higher cost. PPO plans typically offer a greater degree of flexibility and offer more options than others available, although premiums will usually be at an increased rate (Grant, 2022).

Furthermore, a **health maintenance organization (HMO)** provides insurance coverage through a network of physicians who are under contract. The plan participants pay a fee, either monthly or annually, and are required to receive services from a primary care physician. The participant will not be able to receive services from a specialist without receiving a referral from a primary care provider. The HMO typically can charge low premiums and usually a very low or even no deductible. Instead, a low-cost copay is charged for each visit to a provider, medical test administered, or prescription that is filled. This minimizes out-of-pocket expenses for patients and their family members. The cost is the greatest advantage of the HMO. The primary disadvantage will be the restrictions on how the plan can be utilized. If a physician is utilized who is out of the network, the patient will be responsible for costs incurred (Hayes, 2022).

A **point-of-service plan (POS)** combines features of the HMO and the PPO. Costs may be low for participants, but the list of providers may be limited. The plan will pay more toward an out-of-network service if the primary care physician makes a referral rather than if the plan participant goes outside of the network without receiving a referral. The plan usually requires a copay but does not require deductible for services supplied in-network. Price is the most significant disadvantage of a POS. Such a plan can be 50% cheaper than PPO plans but 50% more than HMO premiums. Also, the set of providers utilized may be limited. Plan participants can use providers that are out-of-network but should be prepared to pay higher costs and to be responsible for completing the paperwork for the visit (Kagan, 2022).

Integrated Delivery System

In comparison, an **integrated delivery system (IDS)** is a network of health care facilities that is owned by a parent organization. The health systems are designed to provide a wide variety of services and thus may include hospitals, clinics, ambulatory surgery centers, and imaging centers. The IDS aligns incentives and resources better than most health care delivery systems and thus can improve medical care while also keeping costs under control (Definitive Healthcare, 2023). Al-Saddique (2018) noted that IDSs may be integrated with horizontally or vertically. Horizontal integration means that activities are coordinated across operating units that deliver services at the same level. Vertical integration, in comparison, means that activities are coordinated across operating units that are delivering services at different levels. Al-Saddique indicated that several advantages were possible as a result of the IDS being utilized correctly:

- Increased collaboration: Because IDS implementation requires teamwork, duplication of services is reduced.
- Improved efficiency: Since health care waste is reduced, the quality of care is enhanced.
- Integrated systems: Hospital systems are provided with multiple monitoring and enforcement tools.
- Payer partnerships: As the quality of patient care improves and costs are reduced, hospitals' reputations also improve.
- Improved care management: Care management improves as organizations become more clinically integrated.
- Patient-centered communication: Since IDS emphasizes timely and clear communication, good communication tends to develop among the caregivers, patient, and family members.

Self-Directed Services

Another method of health care delivery is that of **self-directed services**. This typically applies to Medicaid services and means that participants have decision-making authority over certain services and take direct responsibility to manage their services with a support system. The use of self-direction promotes the use of control over the delivery of services through waiver and state plans, including who provides services and how services are provided. An example of this is that participants are given the authority to recruit, hire, train, and supervise the individuals who furnish them services (Medicaid, 2022).

Telehealth

The method of health care delivery that has emerged most significantly as a result of the COVID19 pandemic is **telehealth**. Through the practice of telehealth, the nurse uses video-conferencing to communicate with the patient and remote home patient monitoring to collect clinical data such as blood pressure readings. Rutledge and Gustin (2021) indicate that the nurse who utilizes telehealth:

- Promotes patient wellness
- Provides care in rural or disadvantaged settings
- Manages chronic conditions
- Provides transition of care
- Supports end-of-life care

As the COVID-19 pandemic intensified, telehealth also exploded as the primary health care delivery system being utilized. However, challenges were encountered with implementation of this system. For example, as facilities raced to purchase to purchase equipment to implement telehealth, nurses struggled to cope with delivering health care by this method without having sufficient time for adequate training. Patients were sometimes unhappy with the system since sufficient time had not been allowed to educate regarding privacy concerns or unique cultural concerns. However, as the pandemic began to cool in intensity, nurses adapted to these challenges, and best practices for telehealth began to be developed (Rutledge & Gustin, 2021).

▶ Summary of Key Points in Chapter

The chapter discussed the various health care delivery systems being utilized in the United States. Various types of managed care organizations were compared and contrasted, including the EPO plan, the PPO, the HMO, and POS. Managed care organizations were compared with the IDS and self-directed services. Finally, telehealth as a health care delivery system was discussed along with its relationship to the COVID-19 pandemic.

▶ Conclusion

As was previously mentioned, the COVID-19 pandemic greatly impacted all aspects of the American health care delivery system. Because of it, telehealth began to be implemented by many primary care providers in an attempt to maintain as much personal contact with patients as possible. As the pandemic continues to progress and diminish, it remains to be seen if telehealth will remain at the forefront of health care delivery in the United States or if a more traditional approach will be resumed.

Along with a pandemic, natural and manmade disasters can definitely affect health care delivery as services in every area are interrupted indefinitely. Disaster preparedness for nurses will be discussed in the subsequent chapter.

▶ Critical Thinking Questions

1. Compare and contrast the benefits and disadvantages of:

    a. Exclusive provider organization plans and preferred provider organizations

b. Health maintenance organizations and point-of-service organizations

c. Integrated delivery system and self-directed services

d. Exclusive provider organization plans and telehealth

2. Explain to a patient the requirement of paying a deductible.

3. Explain the advantages of an integrated delivery system. What would you consider to be the primary disadvantages of this system?

4. Explain the advantages of self-directed services. What would you consider to be the primary disadvantages of these services?

5. Explain the advantages of telehealth. What would you consider to be the primary disadvantages of this system?

▶ Scenarios

1. You are a nurse case manager working with a primary care provider who has a large practice. You are working with several patients who will need to change their health care delivery system because changes in the economy. As the nurse case manager, how would you explain to a patient who does not work in any area of health care:

   a. how an exclusive provider organization plan functions?

   b. what a deductible is?

c. what a preferred provider is?

d. how a health maintenance organization functions?

e. how an integrated delivery system functions?

f. how a point-of-service plan functions?

g. how a preferred provider organization functions?

h. how self-directed services function?

i. how telehealth functions?

▶ NCLEX-Style Review Questions

1. You are helping a patient understand the functioning of the integrated delivery system that will be used to deliver his health care services. You explain to the patient that advantages of an integrated delivery system include: (*select all that apply*):
   a. increased collaboration among providers
   b. decreased need for monitoring of hospital systems
   c. improved patient-centered communication
   d. improved care management
   e. increase in provider costs
   f. decreased use of hospital enforcement tools

2. You are a case manager for a primary care provider with a large practice. You recognize that as a result of the COVID-19 pandemic, the health care delivery system that has expanded the most is:
   a. the preferred provider organization
   b. self-directed services
   c. the health maintenance organization
   d. telehealth
   e. the point-of-service plan

3. You are helping a patient understand the functioning of a health maintenance organization. You explain that the primary advantage of such a health care delivery system consists of:
   a. utilization
   b. cost
   c. provider network
   d. documentation

4. You are helping a patient understanding the functioning of a point-of-service plan. You explain that the major disadvantages of such a health care delivery can include: (*select all that apply*)
   a. utilization
   b. cost
   c. provider network
   d. documentation

5. You are working with a health care consumer who is receiving Medicaid. Which health care delivery system is the client most likely to be utilizing?
   a. the preferred provider organization
   b. self-directed services
   c. the health maintenance organization
   d. telehealth
   e. the point-of-service plan

6. You are working with a health care consumer who is receiving health care services through an integrated delivery system that coordinates activities across operating units that are delivering services at different levels. This is commonly known as:
   a. vertical integration
   b. linear integration
   c. horizontal integration
   d. transverse integration

7. You are working with a health care consumer who is receiving health care services through an integrated delivery system that coordinates activities across operating units that are delivering services at the same level. This is commonly known as:
   a. vertical integration
   b. linear integration
   c. horizontal integration
   d. transverse integration

▶ Case Study

You are working as a nurse with an oncologist who has a large practice. You are working with Jim, another nurse who has 12 years of experience. During a weekly group meeting, the director of nursing announces that the practice will be implementing telehealth within the next weeks. You stop for a cup of coffee with Jim. He looks depressed. He tells you, "I just don't understand this telehealth business. I'm working with Mr. Williams, who is a 62-year-old with terminal lung cancer. He has a wife, four grown kids, and three grandkids and was planning to take his wife on a cruise next year until his diagnosis. The doctor doesn't think he'll last until May to see his granddaughter graduate from high school. How is telehealth going to make any difference to him?" What would you say to Jim regarding the benefits of telehealth?

1. Highlight the area in the scenario that corresponds to the primary benefit of telehealth for this patient.
   a. The primary benefit of telehealth for this patient will be ______________.
   b. ____ promotion of his wellness
   c. ____ support of end-of-life care for him
   d. ____ provision of transition of care to another setting
   e. ____ management of chronic disease processes
   f. ____ provision of care in a disadvantaged setting

Concept Map

Create a concept map that is reflective of Mr. Williams' situation.

Note Taker

I. Managed care organizations

A. Exclusive provider organization plan

1. Advantages

2. Disadvantages

B. Preferred provider organization

1. Preferred providers

2. Deductible

3. Advantages

4. Disadvantages

C. Health maintenance organization

1. Advantages

2. Disadvantages

D. Point-of-service organizations

1. Advantages

2. Disadvantages

E. Integrated delivery system

1. Advantages

2. Disadvantages

F. Self-directed services

1. Advantages

2. Disadvantages

G. Telehealth

1. Advantages

References

Al-Saddique, A. (2017). Integrated delivery systems (IDSs) as a means of reducing costs and improving healthcare delivery. *Journal of Healthcare Communications*, *3*(1). https://doi.org/10.4172/2472-1654.100129

Cockerham, W., & Hinote, B. (2008). United States, health system of. In H. K. Heggenhougen (Ed.), *International encyclopedia of public health* (pp. 434–440). Academic Press. https://doi.org/10.1016/B978-012373960-5.00322-1.

Definitive Healthcare. (2023). *Integrated delivery network*. https://www.definitivehc.com/resources/glossary/integrated-delivery-network

Gordon, D. (2021, July 1). *What is an exclusive provider organization plan?* HealthCareInsider.com. https://healthcareinsider.com/exclusive-provider-organization-plan-196923

Grant, M. (2022, March 9). *Preferred provider organization*. Investopedia.com. https://www.investopedia.com/terms/p/preferred-provider-organization.asp

Hayes, A. (2022, March 3). *Health maintenance organization*. Investopedia.com. https://www.investopedia.com/terms/h/hmo.asp

Heaton J, & Tadi P. (2021, March). *Managed care organization*. In: StatPearls [Internet]. StatPearls Publishing.

Kagan, J. (2022, March 10). *Point-of-service (POS) plan*. Investopedia.com. https://www.investopedia.com/terms/p/pointofservice-plan-pos.asp

Medicaid.gov. (n.d.). *Self-directed services*. https://www.medicaid.gov/medicaid/long-term-services-supports/self-directed-services/index.html

Rutledge, C., & Gustin, T. (2021). Preparing nurses for roles in telehealth: Now is the time! *OJIN: The Online Journal of Issues in Nursing*, *26*(1). https://doi.org/10.3912/ojin.vol26no01man03

PART IV

Current Issues in Health Care Delivery

CHAPTER

17

Disaster Preparedness

CHAPTER OBJECTIVES

Upon completion of the chapter, you will be able to:

1. Discuss the American Nurses Association's suggestion for preparing for disasters
2. Describe the Association of Women's Health, Obstetric, and Neonatal Nursing's (AWHONN) guidelines to be applied prior to, during, and after a disaster
3. Discuss Federal Emergency Management Agency's (FEMA) stages of emergency management
4. Analyze recommendations for preparing the nursing workforce for future disasters

KEY TERMS

mitigation

preparedness

response

recovery

Nurses play a vital role in both preparing for imminent disasters and in responding to disasters, as has been shown by the evolving COVID-19 pandemic. The American Nurses Association (ANA) has recognized the strong relationship between nurses and the public who expects that nurses along with other health care providers will respond to their needs when disaster strikes (ANA, 2022). During the recent pandemic, nurses were called upon to care for critically ill patients for lengthy periods of time even as their colleagues and family members were succumbing to the virus. The ANA has indicated that nurses have an ethical obligation to not only care for the public but also to care for themselves (ANA, 2022).

What can nurses do to be as prepared as possible for the inevitable disasters to come, whether natural in nature or manmade? The ANA's suggestions include the following:

- Be aware of employers' emergency response plans.
- Be aware of state and local disaster preparedness and response efforts that are occurring in the area.
- Volunteer with a disaster registry or with the American Red Cross to ensure that they will be properly trained to respond (ANA, 2022).

The Association of Women's Health, Obstetric, and Neonatal Nursing (AWHONN) addressed the need for "all hazards preparedness" in its official position statement that discussed the role of the nurse in emergency preparedness (2012). It developed a series of guidelines designed to be applied prior to, during, and after some type of disastrous event. Although the guidelines were developed prior to the recent pandemic and were initially developed to apply to facilities that offer care to women and infants, they have been adapted here to be applied to any disastrous situation.

Stages of Disaster Preparedness

Prior to the Disaster, Staff Should:

- Ensure that evacuation plans have been developed and are reviewed frequently
- Ensure that an emergency preparedness checklist has been prepared and is reviewed frequently so that supplies can be replaced as needed
- Ensure that strategies for maintaining patient and employee hydration, nutrition, and safe and hygienic accommodations have been developed and are reviewed
- Ensure that a method of obtaining and maintaining patient records in the event of completion loss of electrical grid is in place
- Ensure that emergency measures to provide patient medications and to continue to supply materials for patient procedures such as emergency surgeries are in place

During the Disaster, Staff Should:

- Continue accurate documentation and recordkeeping
- Ensure that the safety of patients and employees is maintained
- Implement strategies to maintain patients and employees in the facility for as long as necessary

After the Disaster, Staff Should:

- Provide mental health support for patients, their family members, and employees
- Reestablish the facility's presence in the community as a health care provider
- Ensure continuity of care
- Reestablish existing infrastructure (AWHONN, 2011)

TABLE 17.1. AWHONN's Stages of Disaster Preparedness

PRIOR TO THE DISASTER	DURING THE DISASTER	AFTER THE DISASTER
Ensure that evacuation plans have been developed and are reviewed frequently	Continue accurate documentation and recordkeeping	Provide mental health support for patients, their family members and employees
Ensure that an emergency preparedness checklist has been prepared and is reviewed frequently	Ensure that safety of patients and employees is maintained	Reestablish the facility's presence in the community as a health care provider

(continued on next page)

PRIOR TO THE DISASTER	DURING THE DISASTER	AFTER THE DISASTER
Ensure that strategies for maintaining patient and employee hydration, nutrition, and safe and hygienic accommodations have been developed and are reviewed	Implement strategies to maintain patients and employees in the facility for as long as necessary	Ensure continuity of care Reestablish existing infrastructure
Ensure that a method of obtaining and maintaining patient records in the event of completion loss of electrical grid is in place		
Ensure that emergency measures to provide patient medications and to continue to supply materials for patient procedures such as emergency surgeries are in place		

Additional lessons in disaster preparedness were derived from the recent COVID-19 pandemic. The nursing workforce changed significantly as a result of implementation of telehealth. As previously stringent regulations relaxed to allow telehealth to be accessible to more patients in a more extensive locale than ever before, it became obvious that nurses could utilize telehealth to appropriately assess patients, monitor symptoms, and provide patient education. As the pandemic progressed, it became obvious that telehealth could be used effectively during a state of emergency to provide health care to patients without spreading the disease process (Chan et al., 2021). Weigel et al. (2020) developed a series of recommendations to continue to expand access to telemedicine in an attempt to be as prepared as possible when disaster strikes again. They suggested:

- Ensuring that the reimbursement of a health insurer to a provider for the diagnosis, consultation, or treatment of the patient via telehealth be expanded to encourage clinicians to utilize this model of care
- Ensuring that patients are able to access telemedicine from their homes to further prevent spreading of contagious disease processes
- Allow use of audio-only telephones for telemedicine appointments since many patients may not have live-video technology
- Invest in telecommunications infrastructure for areas having sites of care that have fewer resources
- Ensure that patients in rural areas have sufficient Internet access to access care

Other lessons in disaster preparedness for nurses that were derived from the pandemic centered around the need to prepare the national nursing workforce overall. A report prepared for

Johns Hopkins's Bloomberg School of Public Health's Center for Health Security found that the national nursing workforce did not feel sufficiently prepared to cope with a disaster such as the COVID-19 pandemic. The authors of the Johns Hopkins report developed recommendations in response to the myriad of forces that were exerting pressure on the nursing workforce at this time. The recommendations included:

- The U.S. Department of Health and Human Services should analyze federal preparedness and response strategies to identify nurses' roles and responsibilities during a pandemic. A plan should be developed to allow nurses to train for these roles.
- Each federal agency's capacity for advancing the emergency preparedness and response knowledge base in the nursing workforce should be identified. This information should be passed on to key stakeholders.
- Accrediting healthcare entities should determine if a facility has sufficient resources to increase the nursing workforce drastically during a pandemic or similar disaster.
- Accrediting health care entities should include education for nurses on pandemic preparedness as a specific requirement.
- The Human Resources and Services Administration should fund nursing workforce development for public health emergency preparedness.
- The Centers for Disease Control and Prevention should fund a National Center for Disaster Nursing and Public Health Emergency Response to provide education and training, career development, and opportunities to network for nurse scientists who are early in their careers.
- Schools of nursing should develop metrics to evaluate nurse preparedness. Such metrics should be implemented across life-long learning programs.
- The American Association of Colleges of Nursing should release revised curriculum *Essentials* and a toolkit for schools of nursing to facilitate the inclusion of emergency preparedness into all existing programs.
- Hospitals should include nurses in emergency preparedness drills and exercises.
- Hospitals should try to establish and maintain crisis leadership skills in managers and executives.

Ultimately, how prepared can nurses be for the disasters, whether natural or manmade, that seem to be inevitable in modern society? The answers may be derived from the Federal Emergency Management Agency (FEMA) stages of emergency management:

Stages of Emergency Management

- **Mitigation:** This includes preventing future emergencies. At this stage, nurses act to protect patients and the facility by decreasing risks and consequences from a disaster.

The main goal is to prevent patient injuries and property damage. Mitigation occurs when nurses serve on a hospital committee that discusses renovations that need to be made to patient rooms to decrease patient falls.

- **Preparedness:** This includes taking actions ahead of time to be prepared for an emergency. Preparedness occurs when nurses who work in an area that experiences frequent hurricanes provide and participate in education, drills, and training that will ensure that staff and patients know how to evacuate if necessary and move to safety.
- **Response:** This includes protecting people and property in the immediate aftermath of a disaster. This occurs when nurses activate the disaster plan to get patients and staff out of harm's way and assist them to evacuate. The success of this stage depends in large measure on the preparation implemented in the earlier stages.
- **Recovery:** This includes restoring normal operating procedures back to normal. This will occur when nurses serve on a hospital committee to rebuild structures damaged in a hurricane, reestablish stakeholder and vendor partnerships after communication is restored, and reduce the facility's vulnerability to storm damage in the future.

▶ Summary of Key Points in Chapter

The chapter discussed aspects of disaster preparedness for nurses. The American Nurses Association's suggestions for preparation for disasters were discussed and compared to the AWHONN's guidelines to be applied prior to, during, and after an imminent disaster. The FEMA stages of emergency management were analyzed along with recommendations for preparing the nursing workforce for future disasters.

▶ Conclusion

Like most Americans, nurses became more concerned than ever regarding disaster preparedness with the advent of the COVID-19 pandemic. Our motivation, as always, continues to be to provide the highest-quality patient care possible in every type of situation, including disasters. However, a challenge to providing high-quality patient care is having sufficient members of the nursing workforce available. The current state of the nursing workforce will be discussed in the subsequent chapter.

▶ Critical Thinking Questions

1. Think about a current or previous workplace. Develop a simple evaluation plan for your facility, including the administrative areas and at least one patient care floor.

2. Think about a current or previous workplace. What would you choose to include in an emergency preparedness checklist for this area?

3. You are responsible for developing a policy on maintaining patient nutrition during a disaster for your facility. Think about what you would include in this policy; also develop strategies for implementing the policy.

4. You are working in a health care facility that has completely lost its electrical grid during a snowstorm. The facility has been using electronic health records for several years. Consider what type of procedure you would implement to move the facility to immediate use of paper records in this emergency. Once the emergency is past and the electrical grid has been restored, how will you commit the temporary paper records to the electronic health records?

5. Think about your own community. If a disaster struck in the area, which agencies do you view as needing to participate in the emergency management plan?

    a. Also discuss the role of each of the agencies. For example, which agencies would be responsible for ensuring that the community water and food supply stay uncontaminated? Which agencies would be responsible for sheltering and protecting displaced persons in the community who need to locate family members?

▶ Scenarios

1. You are a school nurse in an elementary school that has been struck by a tornado. The school is in a suburban area and 10 miles away from a major hospital, which also sustained major damage in the storm. The school is located 25 miles away from a major undamaged hospital. The school serves children ages 5 (kindergarten) to 12 (sixth grade). You have not been seriously injured. As you triage one child after another, what do you consider to be the most important information that you would try to assess regarding each child in this situation?

2. You need to organize the evacuation of the children from the school discussed in question 1. Think about the procedure that you would utilize to evacuate children, both injured and uninjured, from the school discussed in question 1.

3. After the disaster of the school being struck by the tornado, you recognize that mental health counseling should be provided. Identify everyone who will most likely need to be provided access to this. Be sure to consider everyone associated with the disaster, including family members and community members.

4. What do you view as the various ethical issues that would be applicable during a disaster? Think about issues such as patient abandonment, allocation of limited resources, and end-of-life care.

NCLEX-Style Review Questions

1. According to the AWHONN, an appropriate intervention for a nurse to carry out prior to a disaster would be: (*select all that apply*)
   a. ensure that a method of obtaining and maintaining patient records in the event of completion loss of electrical grid is in place
   b. ensure that safety of patients and employees is maintained
   c. ensure that emergency measures to provide patient medications are in place
   d. implement strategies to maintain patients and employees in the facility for as long as necessary
   e. provide mental health support for patients, their family members, and employees
   f. ensure continuity of care

2. According to the AWHONN, an appropriate intervention for a nurse to carry out during a disaster would be: (*select all that apply*)
   a. ensure that a method of obtaining and maintaining patient records in the event of completion loss of electrical grid is in place
   b. ensure that safety of patients and employees is maintained
   c. ensure that emergency measures to provide patient medications are in place
   d. implement strategies to maintain patients and employees in the facility for as long as necessary
   e. provide mental health support for patients, their family members, and employees
   f. ensure continuity of care

3. According to the AWHONN, an appropriate intervention for a nurse to carry out after a disaster would be to: (*select all that apply*)
   a. ensure that a method of obtaining and maintaining patient records in the event of completion loss of electrical grid is in place
   b. ensure that safety of patients and employees is maintained
   c. ensure that emergency measures to provide patient medications are in place
   d. implement strategies to maintain patients and employees in the facility for as long as necessary
   e. provide mental health support for patients, their family members, and employees
   f. continue accurate documentation and record keeping

Match the characteristics with the correct FEMA stage of emergency management.

4. ____protecting patients and the facility by decreasing risks and consequences from a disaster

5. ____nurses serve on a committee to reestablish vendors after communication is restored

6. ____activating the disaster plan to get patients and staff out of harm's way and to evacuate

7. ____nurses serve on a committee to reduce facility's vulnerability to future storm damage

8. ____ nurses participate in drills to ensure that staff and patients know how to evacuate

9. ____ nurses serve on a committee regarding changes to patient rooms to prevent falls

10. ____ nurses serve on a committee to rebuild structures damaged in a storm
    a. Mitigation
    b. Preparedness
    c. Response
    d. Recovery

▶ Case Study

You are working the 7 p.m.–7 a.m. shift on a 40-bed neurology floor tonight. One of your colleagues is Joe. He recently moved to your community after working for 10 years as a nurse in his hometown approximately 50 miles away. The hospital where he previously worked was destroyed in a fire while he was on duty.

About 2 a.m. the pace slows enough for you to stop to get a cup of coffee in the break room. Joe walks in about the same time, and you invite him to sit down with you. He begins to talk about how different this hospital is from his previous 75-bed rural hospital. He tells you about the night when the fire started. "It was so terrible," he says. "I kept running back in trying to get patients out, we all did. There were so many that we couldn't save. There were so many of my colleagues that got hurt, too. I got burned, but not too bad. There were people working in there that I grew up with that died in that fire. I used to want to start working day shift instead of nights. Not now. I can't sleep; I just see the scenes from the fire over and over." Joe seems embarrassed that he has talked about the fire as much as he has and walks out abruptly.

1. Highlight the section in the scenario that corresponds to FEMA's response phase of the emergency management process.

2. Highlight the section in the scenario that would indicate that the "After the Disaster" phase of AWHONN's Stages of Disaster Preparedness has not been fully implemented.

3. Joe participates in drills to learn how to efficiently evacuate patients in the event of a disaster. This corresponds to the ____________ phase of the FEMA stages of emergency management.
    a. mitigation
    b. preparedness
    c. response
    d. recovery

4. What can you do to try to help Joe after his experience in this disaster?

▶ Concept Map

Develop a concept map that illustrates Joe's situation.

▶ Note Taker

I. Preparing for disaster

A. ANA suggestions

B. AWHONN guidelines

1. Prior to the disaster

2. During the disaster

3. After the disaster

II. Lessons learned from the pandemic

A. Implementation of telehealth

B. Preparation of the national nursing workforce

III. FEMA stages of emergency management

A. Mitigation

B. Preparedness

C. Response

D. Recovery

References

American Nurses Association. (n.d.). *Disaster Preparedness.* https://www.nursingworld.org/practice-policy/project-firstline/on-the-go-resource/disaster-preparedness/#Disaster-Preparedness-Basics

Association of Women's Health, Obstetric, and Neonatal Nursing. (2012). The role of the nurse in emergency preparedness. *Journal of Obstetric, Gynecologic & Neonatal Nursing, 41*(2), 322–324. https://doi.org/10.1111/j.1552-6909.2011.01338.x

Chan, G., Bitton, J., Allgeyer, R., Elliott, D., Hudson, L., & Moulton, B. P. (2021, May 31). The impact of COVID-19 on the nursing workforce: A national overview. *OJIN: The Online Journal of Issues in Nursing,* 26(2), Manuscript 2.

Federal Emergency Management Agency. (n.d.) *Emergency management in the United States.* https://training.fema.gov/emiweb/downloads/is111_unit%204.pdf

Veenema, T., Meyer, D., Bell, S., Couig, M., Friese, C., Lavin, R., Stanley, J., Martin, E., Montague, M., Toner, E., Schoch-Spana, M., & Cicero, A. (2020, June 10). *Recommendations for improving national nurse preparedness for pandemic response: Early lessons from COVID-19.* The Johns Hopkins Center for Health Security. https://centerforhealthsecurity.org/2020/new-report-recommendations-for-improving-national-nurse-preparedness-for-pandemic-response-early-lessons-from-covid-19-0.

Weigel, G., Ramaswamy, A., Sobel, L., Salganicoff, A., Cubanski, J., & Free, M. (2020, May 11). *Opportunities and barriers for telemedicine in the U.S. During the COVID-19 emergency and beyond.* Kaiser Family Foundation. https://www.kff.org/womens-health-policy/issue-brief/opportunities-and-barriers-for-telemedicine-in-the-u-s-during-the-covid-19-emergency-and-beyond/.

CHAPTER

18

Nursing Workforce Shortage

CHAPTER OBJECTIVES

Upon completion of the chapter, you will be able to:

1. Discuss the reasons for the current shortage of nurses in the workforce
2. Describe the current shortage of qualified nursing faculty in schools of nursing
3. Discuss the impact of changing demographics in America on the nursing shortage
4. Describe the impact of the COVID-19 pandemic on the existing nursing shortage
5. Analyze the impact of various legislative initiatives on the nursing shortage.

KEY TERMS

Community College and Industry Partnership Grants

Future Advancement of Academic Nursing Act

Graduate Nurse Education pilot

National Health Care Workforce Commission

The recent pandemic focused the public's attention on many areas of health care that needed to be revised or resolved, one of which was the nursing workforce shortage. Despite existing since at least 2010 and undergoing multiple attempts at resolution, the shortage of nurses has only worsened with each successive year. What is the current state of the nursing workforce in America, and why does it continue to exist?

According to the U.S. Bureau of Labor Statistics (BLS), employment of registered nurses is projected to grow 9% from 2020 to 2030. Prior to the pandemic, the BLS projected a shortage of 194,500 openings per year for nurses. The American Nurses Association (2021) indicated that the increased number of nurses needed is attributable to:

- The increased access to health care services for all people because of the Affordable Care Act
- Increased focus on primary care, prevention, wellness, and the management of chronic disease processes
- The complex health care needs of the aging baby-boomer population
- Increased focus on community-based care

However, is this truly indicative of the reasons why nurses are fleeing the bedside?

Why Are Nurses Leaving Bedside Nursing?

According to a survey of almost 1,500 nurses conducted for nurse.org, 36% of nurses reported needing safe staffing, safer patient ratio assignments, and increased pay in order to remain in their current position. Nurses indicated that the need for safe staffing was primarily the reason for their decision to leave their bedside positions (Gaines, 2022).

According to the American Association of Colleges of Nursing (AACN; 2020), there are multiple contributing factors that are impacting the nursing shortage. For example, the AACN has indicated that enrollment in nursing schools is not growing rapidly enough to meet the projected demand for registered nurse and advanced practice registered nurse services. The AACN reported a 5.1% enrollment increase in entry-level baccalaureate program in nursing in 2019. However, this is not sufficient to meet the projected demand for nursing services, including nursing faculty, nurse researchers, and nurses serving as primary care providers.

A related factor is the shortage of qualified nursing school faculty, thus restricting nursing program enrollments. The AACN (2020) has indicated that during the 2019 academic year, U.S. schools of nursing rejected 80,407 qualified applicants from both baccalaureate and graduate nursing programs due to insufficient faculty, clinical sites, classroom space, clinical preceptors, and ultimately lack of funding.

Another factor impacting the current nursing shortage is the changing demographics in America. In 2018, the average age for a registered nurse (RN) was reported to be 50. This is concerning at a time when the U.S. Census Bureau projects that by 2030, the number of U.S. residents ages 65 and older is projected to be approximately 82 million. At a time when there will be larger numbers of people geriatric age who have the typical chronic disease processes associated with older adulthood, there is likely to be fewer numbers of full-time clinical nurses available to provide needed care (AACN, 2020). Bombardieri et al. (2022) indicated that more than one-fifth of the nurses who were polled in 2020 (more than 900,000) indicated that they intended to retire within the next five years.

The already existing nursing shortage has been exacerbated by the COVID-19 pandemic.

According to Bombardieri et al. (2022) chief nursing officers reported vacancy rates for nurses up to 30% throughout the pandemic. Such extensive vacancy rates helped produce an increase in use of travel nurses. Use of travel nursing increased by 35% in 2020 and was expected to increase an additional 40% by the end of 2021. The lucrative pay provided to travel nurses (at times up to four times the usual rate) encouraged nurses who were already exhausted from long hours during the pandemic to leave their usual positions.

Improving the Current Nursing Shortage

What can be done to help resolve the current nursing shortage? Bombardieri et al. (2022) have indicated that higher education is critical to resolution of the shortage. However, there are three primary constraints that will prevent nursing programs from graduating additional nurses: a shortage of qualified nursing faculty, a lack of clinical placement for nursing students, and insufficient campus facilities and equipment. Along with a lack of clinical placements has been a lack of nurse preceptors. These nurses will supervise one to two senior-level nursing students who are beginning to transition into professional practice as they near graduation. Preceptors are not paid, and during the pandemic nurses have been so overworked that they have been unable to assume the extra responsibility of supervision of student nurses.

The existing shortage of nursing faculty has also been exacerbated by the pandemic. As teaching conditions began to be more challenging, including lack of clinical placements for students, dwindling financial resources, and a complete shift to online learning during the months when the pandemic was at its peak, faculty began to be drawn away by the increased pay offered to nursing who worked in any clinical areas. Nursing faculty surveyed during this time reported decreased satisfaction with their jobs, citing low pay as well as the increased workload that is comes with classroom teaching as well as the research, publishing, maintaining their clinical license, and earning promotion and tenure (Bombardieri et al. 2022).

As previously mentioned, hand in hand with a lack of qualified preceptors goes an inadequate number of clinical placements. As health care has moved out of the traditional hospital setting, it has moved into settings such as public health departments, local clinics, and nursing homes. Some of the clinical needs have been filled with the use of simulation. As overwhelmed and overcrowded hospitals shut their doors to nursing students during the pandemic, state boards of nursing granted nursing programs the ability to replace a specific percentage of clinical hours with virtual simulation. Although this has been a short-term remedy to fill some of the required clinical hours, use of simulation requires state-of-the art equipment, including expensive software and mannequins, as well as training for faculty. Also, can simulation provide not just an excellent learning opportunity but a complete substitution in place of clinical experience with a living patient? This remains to be seen post-pandemic (Bombardieri et al., 2022).

Once a clear snapshot of the current state of the nursing shortage has been revealed, potential solutions can be considered. Bombardieri et al. 2022 discussed several pieces of legislation that could improve the situation if passed. The Future Advancement of Academic Nursing Act would award competitive grants to nursing schools to enhance nursing education programs and expand their capacity to respond to public health emergencies such as the pandemic. It would prioritize colleges and universities that serve minorities and also regions with low numbers of medical professionals. This legislation could increase the hiring and recruitment of diverse faculty.

Another piece of legislation that could have a substantial effect on the nursing workforce would be the Community College and Industry Partnership Grants program, which was proposed in the Build Back Better Act. This would make $2 billion available for increasing workforce training in high-demand areas that include nursing. This would allow community colleges to purchase specialized equipment such as the type needed for a simulation laboratory and to improve programs that would enable community college students to transfer to four-year universities while decreasing tuition cost (Bombardieri et al., 2022).

A program that would be helpful if reinstated would be the Graduate Nurse Education pilot, which was originally funded in 2010 as part of the Patient Protection and Affordable Care Act. This allowed the Centers for Medicare & Medicaid Services (CMS) to pay hospitals to increase their clinical education slots and select more advanced practice registered nurses than usual. Another helpful program would be the National Health Care Workforce Commission, which was originally authorized by the Affordable Care Act in 2010. Although members of the commission were appointed, funding was never appointed. If the National Health Care Workforce Commission was both fully staffed and funded, it could work with health care workforce professionals, colleges and universities, researchers, and government agencies and advise on the state of the nursing workforce shortage, particularly during times of great demand, such as the recent pandemic (Bombardieri et al., 2022).

▶ Summary of Key Points in Chapter

The chapter discussed the reasons for the current shortage of nurses in the workforce. The current shortage of qualified nursing faculty in schools of nursing was also described along with the impact of changing demographics in America on the nursing shortage. Finally, the impact of the COVID-19 pandemic on the existing nursing shortage was analyzed along with the potential impact of various legislative initiatives on the nursing shortage.

▶ Conclusion

Ultimately, what can the average nurse do to contribute to resolution of the current nursing shortage? Make certain that you are in the nursing workforce, whether at the bedside in patient care or as faculty in a school of nursing and remain in the workforce despite the difficulties that were spotlighted by the pandemic. Also, become politically active so that you have a voice in the development of your own profession's workforce.

▶ Critical Thinking Questions

1. Think about the various factors that were discussed pertaining to the current shortage of nursing faculty in schools of nursing. What do you consider to be the one factor that is influencing this situation the most? Be prepared to support your answer with accurate information.

2. Consider the changing demographics in America. Which one do you consider to be exerting the greatest effect on the current nursing shortage? Be prepared to support your answer with accurate information.

3. Consider the various pieces of legislation that were discussed in this chapter. Which one do you view as making the greatest impact on the current shortage of nursing faculty if it were passed? Be prepared to support your answer with accurate information.

4. The American Nurses Association discussed various factors that the organization views as affecting the nursing shortage. Explain how the increased access to health care services for all people because of the Affordable Care Act contributed to the nursing shortage.

5. The American Nurses Association discussed various factors that the organization views as affecting the nursing shortage. Explain how the increased focus on primary care, prevention, wellness, and the management of chronic disease processes contributed to the nursing shortage.

6. The American Nurses Association discussed various factors that the organization views as affecting the nursing shortage. Explain how the complex health care needs of the aging baby boomer population contributed to the nursing shortage.

7. The American Nurses Association discussed various factors that the organization views as affecting the nursing shortage. Explain how the increased focus on community-based care contributed to the nursing shortage.

▶ Scenarios

1. You are a nurse recruiter for a large metropolitan hospital (700 beds). What strategies would you implement to hire qualified nurses to fill the open positions in this facility?

2. You are a nurse recruiter for a small rural hospital (90 beds). What strategies would you implement to hire qualified nurses to fill the open positions in this facility?

3. You are a nurse recruiter for a home health agency. What strategies would you implement to hire qualified nurses to fill the open positions in this facility?

4. You are a nurse recruiter for a university School of Nursing. The university is located in a major metropolitan city. There are three open faculty positions. What strategies would you implement to hire qualified nurse faculty to fill the open positions in this facility?

5. You are a nurse recruiter for a university School of Nursing. The university is located in a small town in the northeastern United States. There are three open faculty positions. What strategies would you implement to hire qualified nurse faculty to fill the open positions in this facility?

NCLEX-Style Review Questions

1. Benefits of the Future Advancement of Academic Nursing Act include: (*select all that apply*)
   - a. awarding competitive grants to nursing schools to enhance nursing education programs
   - b. making $2 billion available for increasing nurse workforce training in high-demand areas
   - c. would expand nursing schools' capacity to respond to public health emergencies
   - d. would prioritize colleges serving minorities and regions with decreased medical professionals

2. Benefits of the Community College and Industry Partnership Grants program include: (*select all that apply*)
   - a. making $2 billion available for increasing nurse workforce training in high-demand areas
   - b. would allow colleges to purchase specialized equipment such as simulation laboratory
   - c. awarding competitive grants to nursing schools to enhance nursing education programs
   - d. would help college students to transfer to four-year universities while decreasing tuition cost

3. Benefits of the Graduate Nurse Education pilot include which of the following? (*select all that apply*)
   a. It allowed CMS to pay hospitals to increase their clinical education slots
   b. It works with health care professionals, universities, researchers, and government agencies
   c. It advises on state of the nursing workforce shortage, particularly during the recent pandemic
   d. It would allow hospitals to select more advanced practice registered nurses than usual

4. Benefits of the National Health Care Workforce Commission include which of the following? (*select all that apply*)
   a. It allowed CMS to pay hospitals to increase their clinical education slots
   b. It works with health care professionals, universities, researchers, and government agencies
   c. It has advised on the state of the nursing workforce shortage, particularly during the recent pandemic
   d. It would allow hospitals to select more advanced practice registered nurses than usual.

▶ Case Study

You are working the 7 p.m.–7 a.m. shift on a busy 48-bed medical oncology floor. At 1 a.m., you go to the nurse's lounge for a cup of coffee and find Joyce also taking a quick break. She looks exhausted and tells her that this is her fifth 12-hour shift in a row. "Joyce, why would you schedule yourself for so many shifts?" you ask her, horrified.

"They're just so short-handed, "she tells you, "and the nurse manager has been so nice to me that I hated to refuse. But I can't go on like this much longer. I didn't get out of here until 9 a.m. yesterday, and I almost wrecked my car on the way home. I'm desperate to transfer somewhere else. I love the patients and my coworkers, but I can't hold out much longer. I'd love to be able to teach one day, but I've got to have a better schedule than this to go back to school. I just don't know what to do."

1. How could you most effectively advise Joyce?
2. Highlight all of the individual factors that are contributing to the nursing workforce shortage in the case study.

3. One of the most effective things that a nurse can do to contribute to the resolution of the nursing workforce shortage is:
   a. assume a leadership position in the nursing profession
   b. become politically active as a registered nurse
   c. practice self-care by avoiding working overtime
   d. work as many shifts as possible as a nurse

Concept Map

Create a concept map that illustrates Joyce's situation.

Note Taker

1. Why does the current nursing shortage exist?

A. Contributing factors

1. Enrollment in nursing schools

2. Shortage of nursing faculty

3. Changing demographics

4. COVID-19 pandemic

B. Factors unique to nursing schools

1. Lack of clinical placements

2. Insufficient campus facilities and equipment

3. Lack of clinical preceptors

II. Potential solutions to the current nursing shortage

A. Future Advancement of Academic Nursing Act

B. Community College and Industry Partnership Grants

C. Graduate Nurse Education pilot

D. National Health Care Workforce Commission

References

American Association of Colleges of Nursing. (2020). *Fact sheet: nursing shortage*. https://www.aacnnursing.org/Portals/42/News/Factsheets/Nursing-Shortage-Factsheet.pdf

American Nurses Association. (2021, September 1). *ANA urges US Department of Health and Human Services to declare nurse staffing shortage a national crisis*. https://www.nursingworld.org/news/news-releases/2021/ana-urges-us-department-of-health-and-human-services-to-declare-nurse-staffing-shortage-a-national-crisis/

Bombardieri, M., Custer, B., Neal, A., Schweitzer, J., & Zhavoronkova, M. (2022, May 24). How to ease the nursing shortage in America. https://www.americanprogress.org/article/how-to-ease-the-nursing-shortage-in-america/

Gaines, K. (2022, January 26). *What's really behind the nursing shortage? 1500 nurses share their stories*. https://nurse.org/articles/nursing-shortage-study/

CHAPTER

19

Violence in the Workplace

KEY TERMS

workplace violence

workplace incivility

CHAPTER OBJECTIVES

Upon completion of the chapter, you will be able to:

1. Discuss the four different types of workplace violence as defined by the NIOSH
2. Define workplace incivility
3. Discuss federal legislation that may decrease the incidence of workplace violence
4. Describe ways in which hospitals can decrease the incidence of workplace violence
5. Describe ways in which nurses can become a change agent in decreasing workplace violence

Types of Workplace Violence

According to the National Institute for Occupational Safety and Health (NIOSH), workplace violence consists of physically and psychologically damaging actions that occur in a workplace setting. Examples of workplace violence can consist of direct physical assaults with or without weapons, written or verbal threats, physical or verbal harassment, and homicide. According to the NIOSH, workplace violence can be classified into four types:

This involves criminal intent by individuals with no relationship to the workplace or the employees.

Type II: This involves a customer, client, or patient. In this type, a person becomes violent while receiving services from the business.

Type III: This involves worker-on-worker violence and occurs when an employee attacks or threatens another employee.

Type IV: This involves personal relationships. It occurs when the violence is instigated by someone with a personal relationship to the business or one of the employees (American Nurses Association, 2021).

Workplace violence is an unfortunate reality in health care. The exact numbers of violent acts that affect nurses are unknown because most violent acts go unreported. The importance of reducing the incidence of workforce violence is emphasized by the consequences of such violent acts. They lead to a decreased commitment to nursing and the health care organization, an increase in absenteeism, and a decrease in the quality of teamwork and health care being provided. Kvas and Seljak (2014) noted that the greatest effects of workforce violence are felt by the victim. They include negative effects on the victim's health, dissatisfaction with the victim's life and work, a decrease in confidence, and an increase in emotional exhaustion and burnout. They noted that victims frequently do not report the violent acts because they believe that reporting the incident wouldn't change anything. Some victims also fear losing their job as a result of reporting the violent act (Kvas & Seljak, 2014).

Findorff et al. (2005) found that a health care employee is more likely to report the perpetrator of a violent act in the workplace when:

- The nurse told the perpetrator to stop but the perpetrator escalated the situation
- Lost work time resulted from the incident
- There was an increased frequency in both verbal and nonverbal threats of violence
- The incidents involved adverse health symptoms resulting from the violence
- The employee used the employee assistance program after the incident
- The employee had to use the health care system to treat the results of the violence

Workplace Incivility

An offshoot of workplace violence is **workplace incivility**. Warner et al. (2016) have defined this phenomenon as repeated incidents of intimidation or abusive behavior, including the abuse of power and the levying of unfair sanctions. These incidents will cause the recipient to feel humiliated and threatened. Like workplace violence, workplace incivility is frequently underreported. It is estimated that up to 85% of nurses experience some form of workplace incivility. Warner et al. (2016) have indicated that an uncivil work environment contributes significantly to nurse turnover and that the average hospital will spend an estimated $379,500 for each percentage of increase in nursing staff turnover. Most importantly, workplace incivility can jeopardize patient safety. For example, nurses may carry out a questionable of unsafe practice rather than ask a colleague known to practice incivility for assistance or clarification. Recognizing this, in 2009, The Joint Commission implemented standards that would require health care leaders to maintain a culture of safety, which includes a lack of tolerance for workplace incivility (Warner et al., 2016).

Once the current state of workplace violence and workplace incivility is revealed, the question becomes: Can this situation be changed successfully? Jones (2021) noted that help may come in the form of federal legislation. In 2021, the House of Representatives passed the Workplace Violence Prevention for Health Care and Social Workers Act. The bill requires the Occupational Safety and Health Administration (OSHA) to create enforceable safety standards by 2025. Although the American Association of Colleges of Nursing (AACN) as well as the Nursing Community Coalition were both in support of the act, the American Hospital Association (AHA) opposed the bill. The AHA asserted that no need for new OSHA standards exists since hospitals have already implemented policies and programs designed to address incidents of workplace violence. The AHA has also expressed concern that the bill's costly requirements will strain the budgets of hospitals serving rural and underserved communities (Jones, 2021).

Preventing Violence Against Health Care Workers

In order to further prevent violence against health care workers, the AACN has urged hospitals to:

- Educate staff on how to recognize the potential for violence, deescalate potentially violent situations, and both prevent and respond appropriately to violence
- Establish a clear and consistent structure for reporting incidences of workplace violence; policies and procedures on how to report violent incidences to law enforcement should be easy to understand and implement
- Encourage employees to bring charges against anyone who assaults a health care worker and be supportive of staff members who choose to press charges
- Assist employees to cope with violent incidents by developing resources and support programs
- Evaluate staffing and patient classification systems that could either contribute or significantly reduce the risk of violence
- Verify that adequate security systems and personnel are being utilized, including alarm systems, emergency response protocols, and highly trained security personnel (Jones, 2021).

Green (2019) indicated the importance of the nurse leader who is employed in a facility that is the site of frequent violent incidents or workplace incivility becoming a change agent. How can this take place? Green recommends initially eliciting feedback from staff and then using self-reflection to analyze your own leadership style. She recommends using the democratic leadership style when addressing workplace incivility since this style allows for objectivity when discussing workplace dysfunction even as multiple views are shared within the group. The democratic leader will use constructive criticism to implement change in the group and to encourage group members to make decisions together. Use of this leadership style will allow team members who are the target of workplace incivility to feel that some type of lasting change for the better will occur in the work facility. Allowing for shared viewpoints will decrease staff members' fear and anxiety while encouraging open discussion. As you collaborate with staff members, you can address the negative behaviors that have been reported to be associated with uncivil conduct. It may be helpful to have a regularly scheduled time to meet with staff members to discuss behavioral expectations, uncivil conduct that has occurred, and the consequences of uncivility. Violence and/or uncivil conduct should never be excused, overlooked, or minimized (see Table 19.1).

TABLE 19.1. How to Become a Change Agent

• Initially elicit feedback from staff
• Use self-reflection to analyze your own leadership style
• Encourage multiple views to be shared within the group
• Allow for shared viewpoints to encourage open discussion
• Have a regularly scheduled time to meet with staff members to discuss behavioral expectations, uncivil conduct that has occurred, and the consequences of uncivility
• Avoid allowing a shortage of nursing staff to cause you to overlook incidents of incivility
• Avoid blaming or identifying the affected individuals in front of other staff members
• If counseling is ineffective, move to progressive discipline

In addition, don't allow a shortage of nursing staff to cause you to overlook incidents of incivility. Remind staff that there is a zero tolerance for such incidents. Avoid blaming or identifying the affected individuals in fr Initiate counseling for the staff member who engages in violence, bullying, or workplace incivility. If counseling is ineffective, move to progressive discipline (2019).

▶ Summary of Key Points in Chapter

The chapter discussed the concept of workplace violence as it pertains to health care and the various types of workplace violence as defined by the NIOSH. Federal legislation that may decrease the incidence of such violence was discussed. Ways in which hospitals can decrease the incidence of workplace violence were delineated. Finally, the chapter discussed ways in which nurses can become a change agent in decreasing the incidence of workplace violence.

▶ Conclusion

Workplace violence and its relative, workplace incivility, are still a reality in health care and particularly in nursing, but the situation can change. Nurses have always been at the forefront of significant change in health care. If the current state of complacent acceptance of workplace violence and incivility as being inevitable in healthcare is to change, nursing must lead the way.

▶ Critical Thinking Questions

1. Consider your current or past work situation or a colleague's work experience. Describe an experience that you are familiar with that is similar to Type I workplace violence as defined by the NIOSH.

2. Consider your current or past work situation or a colleague's work experience. Describe an experience that you are familiar with that is similar to Type II workplace violence as defined by the NIOSH.

3. Consider your current or past work situation or a colleague's work experience. Describe an experience that you are familiar with that is similar to Type III workplace violence as defined by the NIOSH.

4. Consider your current or past work situation or a colleague's work experience. Describe an experience that you are familiar with that is similar to Type IV workplace violence as defined by the NIOSH.

5. You are a prominent nurse leader in your facility and your local community. Develop a presentation that you could give to your state's hospital association arguing in favor of the Workplace Violence Prevention for Health Care and Social Workers Act.

6. Compare and contrast workplace violence with workplace incivility.

Scenarios

1. Lois tells John, her nurse manager, that the new surgeon with the surgical group that sends patients to her floor has been making unwanted advances toward her. Lois indicates that she has let the surgeon know that his advances are unwanted; however, he continues to harass her. She tells John that if she has to, she'll move to a lower-paying job on another shift to get away from the surgeon. Lois is an experienced registered nurse (RN) who is well respected by her colleagues, and John really needs her in her current position of charge nurse.

    a. What should Lois do next?

    b. What should John do regarding this situation?

    c. What should the director of nursing do?

2. Carl and Bill are both RNs who work in the same intensive care unit on the same shift. They have always gotten along well and had an excellent working relationship. However, Carl's wife recently left him and is in the process of divorcing him. Bill has quietly started dating Carl's soon-to-be ex-wife. As Bill arrived to start his shift tonight at the hospital, Carl walked up to his car and began a fight with him in the parking lot. The two nurses are separated by hospital security guards and taken to the director of nursing's office.

    a. What should the director of nursing do about this situation?

    b. What specifically should happen to Bill?

    c. What specifically should happen to Carl?

3. You are the administrator at the hospital where Lois, Carl, and Bill are all employed. You are very concerned when you hear about these employees. You decide that a plan must be implemented to decrease the incidence of workplace violence in your hospital.

    a. What plan would you implement to decrease incidents similar to Lois' situation?

b. What plan would you implement to decrease incidents similar to that of Carl and Bill?

▶ NCLEX-Style Review Questions

1. Two hospital employees begin to shout at each other in the parking deck, and one worker suddenly stabs the other employee. According to the NIOSH, this type of workplace violence is considered to be:
   a. Type I
   b. Type II
   c. Type III
   d. Type IV

2. A person who arrives at the emergency department complaining of shortness of breath becomes upset that he has to wait to be seen by a physician. The patient begins shouting at the unit secretary and demanding to be seen immediately. The unit secretary asks security guards to intervene after the patient begins leaning across the desk and shaking his fist in her face. According to the NIOSH, this type of workplace violence is considered to be:
   a. Type I
   b. Type II
   c. Type III
   d. Type IV

3. A person who has no relationship to any of the patients or the employees is walking through the hallways of a hospital when he suddenly physically assaults a unit clerk for apparently no reason. According to the NIOSH, this type of workplace violence is considered to be:
   a. Type I
   b. Type II
   c. Type III
   d. Type IV

4. Millie is a nurse who is going through a divorce. She arrives to start her shift on her floor and is confronted by her husband, who steps out of the stairwell and starts dragging her down the hall by one arm toward the elevator. "We're going to end this right now!" he says. According to the NIOSH, this type of workplace violence is considered to be:
   a. Type I
   b. Type II
   c. Type III
   d. Type IV

5. Julie is a nurse who occasionally sees Jim, a phlebotomist, in the hallway. One day Jim asks Julie out on a date. Julie, who is happily married, refuses. Jim begins to harass her. This behavior escalates until Jim suddenly grabs Julie and tries to kiss her. What should Julie's initial action be?
   a. Begin documenting information in preparation for litigation
   b. Enroll in the employee assistance program
   c. Notify her nurse manager of the situation
   d. Discuss the incident with hospital security personnel

▶ Case Study

You and Jill have just interviewed for your first nursing positions after graduating from your nursing program. When you ask her how her interview went, Jill looks pale and worried. "The interview was fine," she says, "but I talked to my senior preceptor about that floor after the interview, and she says not to accept the job because it's the worst floor in the hospital. My preceptor said that the nurse manager is really strict and the nurses are so hard to get along with that they can't keep a charge nurse! She says that no nurse ever wants to float to that floor because the nurses won't help each other and they ignore new people. What do you think that I should do?"

1. What advice would you give Jill?
2. Highlight all of the incidences in the case study that you would classify as workforce violence.
3. Highlight all of the incidences in the case study that you would classify as workforce incivility.

4. The registered nurse is working in the emergency department on the night shift when her ex-husband appears unexpectedly and tries to attack her. According to the NIOSH, this is considered to be ______________ workplace violence.
   a. Type I
   b. Type II
   c. Type III
   d. Type IV

▶ Concept Map

Develop a concept map that is centered around Jill's anxiety regarding her new position.

▶ Note Taker

I. Types of workplace violence

A. Type I

B. Type II

C. Type III

D. Type IV

II. Workplace incivility

III. Workplace Violence Prevention for Health Care and Social Workers Act

IV. What can hospitals do to prevent workplace violence?

V. How nurses can function as change agents

References

American Nurses Association. (2021). *Workplace violence.* https://www.nursingworld.org/practice-policy/advocacy/state/workplace-violence2/

Findorff, M., McGovern, P., Wall, M., & Gerberich, S. (2005). Reporting violence to a healthcare employer: A cross-sectional study. *AAOHN Journal, 53*(9), 399–406.

Green, C. (2019). Workplace incivility: Nurse leaders as changes agents. *Nursing Management, 50*(1), 51–53.

Jones, M. (2021). *Preventing workplace violence in healthcare.* https://www.aacn.org/blog/preventing-workplace-violence-in-healthcare

Kvas, A., & Seljak, J. (2014). Unreported workplace violence in nursing. *International Nursing Review, 61*, 344–351. https://doi.org/10.1111/inr.12106

Warner, J., Sommers, K., Zappa, M., & Thornlow, D. (2016). Decreasing workplace incivility. *Nursing Management, 47*(1), 22–30.

Index

A

accommodation, 264
accountability, 251
acculturation, 49, 135
active listening, 231, 233–236
administrative law, 111
advanced directive, 113
advance directives, 113
advanced practice nurses, 14
American Association of Colleges of Nursing (AACN), 14–15, 342
American Hospital Association (AHA), 342
American Nurses Association (ANA), 314
American Nurses Association's (ANA) code of ethics, 93
American Nurses Association's Nursing Hall of Fame, 11
American Red Cross, 9
Army Nurse Corps, 11
assault, 112
assessment, 183–185
  emergency, 184
  focused, 184
  initial, 184
  of patients' spiritual needs, 214
  ongoing, 185–186
assimilation, 135
Association of Women's Health, Obstetric, and Neonatal Nursing (AWHONN), 314
authority, 251
autonomy, 93
avoidance, 264

B

Barton, Clara, 9
battery, 112
bedside nursing, 329
Bellevue Hospital, 11
benchmark, 286
beneficence, 93
Bible, 3
biomedical health view, 138
Bloom's taxonomy, 197
Boston Training School, 11
Brahmanism, 3
Build Back Better Act, 330
Bullwinkel, Vivien, 13
bullying behavior, 264

C

carative factors, 47–48
  balance, 48
  co-create, 48
  deepen, 47
  embrace, 47
  forgive, 47
  inspire, 47
  minister, 48
  nurture, 47
  open, 48
  trust, 47
Catholic Church, 4
causal factors, charting, 287–288
cause-and-effect diagram, 287–288
change agent, becoming, 343
channel of communication, 226–227
Cheney, Ednah Dow, 10
Christianity, 4
civil law, 112–113
Clark, Colonel Mildred, 13
clinical nurse leader (CNL), 15
coercive power, 262
collaboration, 264
communication process, 224
  barriers to, 231–234
  elements, 225
  incongruent communication, 230–231
  modes and channels, 226–227
  nonverbal form, 229–230
  using "I" statements, 237
  verbal form, 227–228
  with aggressive person, 237–238
  with peers, 234–235
  with physicians, 236–237
  with subordinates, 235–236
  with upper-level management, 237–238
Community College and Industry Partnership Grants program, 330
competition, 264
concept mapping, 200–201

conceptual frameworks, 32
confidentiality, 93
conflict
  interpersonal, 264
  resolution, 263–264
  responses to, 263
  role, 261
  stages of progression of, 264
constitutional law, 110
contextual stimuli, 42
contract law, 112
Cornell University-New York Hospital School of Nursing, 10
COVID-19 pandemic, 95, 300, 329
COVID19 pandemic, 14
creativity, 14, 253
Crimean War, 1854, 6
criminal law, 110–111
cultural awareness, 49
cultural diversity, 48
cultural humility, 131–133
culturally congruent care, 49
cultural universality, 48
culture
  cultural-related factors affecting communication, 137–138
  elements, 133
  factors characterizing, 133–134
  functioning as, 134–135
  shock, 134
  subcultures, 134
Cumming, Kate, 9–10

D
Davis, President Jefferson, 10
deaconesses, 4
Deborah, 3
decision-making, 253
deductible, 299
defamation, 112
delegation, 251
  barriers to using, 252
  intervention to an unlicensed person, 252–253
  skills needed to set priorities, 253–254
dependent nursing interventions, 198
diagnosis, 185–197
  absorption, 187
  activity/rest, 188
  body image, 189
  cardiovascular/cardiopulmonary responses, 188
  caregiving roles, 190
  comfort, 193
  communication, 189
  coping/stress tolerance, 190–191
  determining, 196
  digestion, 187
  energy balance, 188
  family relationships, 190
  gastrointestinal function, 187
  growth/development, 194
  hydration, 187
  ingestion, 186
  integumentary function, 187
  life principles, 191–192
  metabolism, 187
  NANDA approved, 186–197
  nutrition, 186–187
  of self-care deficit, 197
  perception/cognition, 189
  process of formulating, 196
  respiratory function, 187–188
  role performance, 190
  role relationship, 189
  safety/protection, 192–193
  self-care, 188
  self-esteem, 189
  self-perception, 189
  sexuality, 190
  sleep, 188
  urinary function, 187
diagnostic operation, 45
diagonal communication, 226
disaster preparedness
  ANA's suggestions, 314
  AWHONN's stages, 315–317
  emergency management, 317–318
discipline of license, 77–79
  abuse, 77–78
  boundary violations, 77–78
  drug-related, 77–78
  fraud, 77, 79
  positive criminal background check, 79–80
  practice-related, 77–78
  sexual misconduct, 77–78
diversity, 131
Dix, Dorothea, 7–8
doctor of nursing practice degree, 14
doctor of nursing practice (DNP), 14
"do not resuscitate" orders, 94
downward communication, 226
durable power of attorney, 113

E
Edwin Smith surgical papyrus, 2–3
electronic health record (EHR), 155–157
  outcomes of use, 156
  use of, 155–156
email, 229–230
  netiquette rules, 230
emergency assessment, 184
emergency management, 317–318
  mitigation, 317

preparedness, 318
recovery, 318
response, 318
energy fields, 40
English military health care, 7
ethical dilemma, 92
ethical issues in nursing, 92
advanced directive, 113
civil law, 112–113
confidentiality, 114
critical care and futile care, conflict between, 96
end-of-life care, 96
ethical decision-making, 93–94
managed care system, 96
moral distress, 95–96
new graduates' expectations and reality, conflict between, 96
physicians and nurses, conflict between, 95–96
related to death and dying, 94–95
use of drugs and alcohol outside workplace, 111
ethnic and racial minorities, 135
ethnicity, 49
etiology, 194
evaluation phase of nursing process, 200–201
exclusive provider organization plan, 298
exclusive provider organization plan (EPO), 298–299
expert power, 262

F

Fairchild, Hedlen, 11–12
false imprisonment, 112
Federal Emergency Management Agency (FEMA), 317
felony, 111
FICA Spiritual History Tool, 213
fidelity, 93
fishbone diagram, 287
5-why analysis, 288
Fliedner, Theodor, 6
Florence Nightingale, 6–7
nursing theory, 32–33
focal stimuli, 42
focused assessment, 184
foreign-born individuals, 137
Fox, Annie G., 12
fraud, 112
French Sisters of Charity, 6
Fuller, Thomas, 5, 7–8
futile care, 95
Future Advancement of Academic Nursing Act, 330

G

Graduate Nurse Education pilot, 330
grapevine, 226

H

Hays, Colonel Anna May, 13
health awareness, 186
health equity, 131, 136–138
Health Insurance Portability and Accountability Act of 1996 (HIPAA), 114, 152, 230
guidelines for telemedicine, 154
penalties for violations of, 153–154
Privacy Rule, 152
Security Rule, 152–154
health maintenance organization, 298
health maintenance organization (HMO), 299
health management, 186
health promotion, 186
Healthy People 2030, 135–136
Henderson, Virginia, 35–37, 43
environment, 36
functions of nurse, 36
health, 36
individual, 36
nursing, 36
Hinduism, 3
holistic health view, 138
horizontal communication, 226

I

immigrants, health status of, 136–137
immunizations, 136
inclusion, 131
incongruent communication, 230–231
independent nursing interventions, 199
Indian historical documents, 3
Indian surgery, 3
informatics, 152
informational power, 262
informed consent, 113
initial assessment, 184
integrated delivery system (IDS), 299–300
horizontal integration, 299–300
vertical integration, 300
interdependent nursing interventions, 199
International Red Cross, 9
intervention phase of nursing process, 198–199
invasion of privacy, 112
I-SBAR-R technique, 235

J

justice, 93

K

King, Imogene, 42–44
environment, 44
health, 44
individual, 43
interpersonal system, 42–43
nursing's goal, 43

personal system, 42
social system, 42
theory of goal attainment, 42–43

L

lateral violence, 264
learning domains
affective, 168, 170
cognitive, 167, 170
psychomotor, 168, 170
learning process, factors affecting, 168–170
legitimate power, 262
Leininger, Madeleine, 48
Levites, 3
licensed practical nurse (LPN), 76
licensure in nursing
categories of disciplinary cases, 77–79
disciplinary actions, 76
evaluation of applictions, 76
issue of licenses, 76
process, 75–77
renewal of licenses, 76
requirements for examination, 76
sustaining discipline of license, 77–79
listening, 229
living will, 113

M

magico-religious health view, 138
Mahoney, Mary Eliza, 11
Malinta Hospital, 13
malpractice, 113
managed care organizations, 298–299
managerial supervision, 273
Maslow's hierarchy of needs, 199
Massachusetts General Hospital, 11
misdemeanor, 111
models, 32
moral courage, 95
moral distress, 95–96
morals, 92
Mosaic Law, 3
mother-child relationship, 2
moving hospital, 11
multistate licensure compact, 111

N

National Association of Colored Graduate Nurses, 11
National Council Licensure Examination (NCLEX) professional licensure examination, 76
National Council of State Boards of Nursing, 76
National Health Care Workforce Commission, 330
National Institute for Occupational Safety and Health (NIOSH), 341
National League for Nursing, 14
National Women's Hall of Fame, 11
Navy Nurse Corps, 11
Navy WAVES, 12
negligence, 113
New England Hospital for Women and Children, 10
nonmaleficence, 93
nontransactional conversation, 235
nonverbal communication, 226, 229–230
North American Nursing Diagnosis Association (NANDA), 185, 196
Nurse Licensure Compact, 77
nurse-patient relationship
exploitation phase, 34
identification phase, 34
nurse's roles in, 35
orientation phase, 34
resolution phase, 34
Nurse Practice Act, 76–77, 111
nursing
during civil war, 7–10
during Vietnam-era, 13–14
during World War I, 11–12
during World War II, 12–13
history, timeline, 16–17
modern, 6–7
origins, 2–4
qualifications for nurses, 5–9
secular, 4–6
Nursing Community Coalition, 342
nursing goal, 197
nursing problems, 195
nursing process, 182–183
advantages of, 183
assessment, 183–185
diagnosis, 185–197
evaluation, 200–201
intervention, 198–199
planning, 197–198
nursing shortage, strategies to improve, 329–330
nursing theory, 31–32
against excessive noise in hospitals, 32
Betty Neuman's, 46–47
clean air and water, sanitation, light, and bathing, 32
Dorothea Orem's, 44–45
environment, 33
Florence Nightingale's, 32–33
health, 34
Hildegard Peplau's, 34–35
Ida Orlando's, 37–39
Imogene King's, 42–44
Jean Watson's, 47–49
Martha Rogers', 39–40
modes of adaptation, 41
nurses, role of, 33

Sister Callista Roy's, 41–42
Virginia Henderson's, 35–37

O

objective data, 185
Occupational Safety and Health Administration (OSHA), 342
ongoing assessment, 184–185
Orem, Dorothea, 44–45
health, 45
human being, 45
nursing problem, 45
theory of nursing, 44–45
Orlando, Ida, 37–39
health, 38
human being, 38
nurse-patient relationship, 37
nurse's perception about patient's behavior, 37–39
nursing, 38
nursing problem, 38
nursing process, 38
theory of nursing, 37–39
outcome criteria, 197–198
outcome measure, 287

P

papyrus, 2
Patient Self-Determination Act, 113
Paula of Actin, 4
peer communication, 234–235
Peplau, Hildegard
nurse's roles in nurse-patient relationship, 35
nursing theory, 34–35
therapeutic interpersonal relationship, 34
performance measurement, 286–287
persuasive power, 262
physicians–nurses communication, 236–237
planning phase of nursing process, 197–198
affective domain, 197
cognitive domain, 197
outcome criteria, 197–198
psychomotor domain, 197
point-of-service organizations, 298
point-of-service plan (POS), 299
power
coercive, 262
expert, 262
informational, 262
legitimate, 262
persuasive, 262
referent, 262
reward, 262
preferred provider organization, 298
preferred provider organization (PPO), 299
preferred providers, 299
prescriptive operations, 45
privacy, 93
problem-solving, 254
processes, 32
process measure, 287
professional judgment, 251, 253
propositions, 32
Protestantism, 4
public law, 110–112

Q

quality improvement in nursing, 286

R

referent power, 262
Reformation, 4
registered nurse (RN), 76–77, 92, 95
average age, 329
communicating with a supervisor, 238
concept of advanced directives, 113
employment of, 328
evaluation, 200
functions, 182
impact of contract, 112
incongruent communication, 230–231
nursing interventions, 199
nursing process, 183
responsibility to maintain confidentiality, 114
transitioning, 131
verbal communication techniques, 228
regulation, 75
regulatory operations, 45
residual stimuli, 42
responsibility, 251
reward power, 262
Richards, Linda, 10–11
Rogers, Edith Nourse, 12
Rogers, Martha, 39–40
role conflict, 95, 261
root cause analysis, 287

S

Seaman, Dr. Valentine, 10
self-care deficit theory, 44
self-directed services, 300
sentinel events, 287–288
silence, 229
Smithsonian Institution, 11
socialization, 134
spiritual assessment, 212–215
spiritual distress, 212
spirituality, 212
spiritual needs, 212
spiritual nursing care behaviors, 214–215
state nurse practice act, 251
Stout, Dr. Samuel, 10

subjective data, 185
supervision, 251, 273
  barriers to effective, 274–276
  development of effective clinical, 274
  managerial, 273
  personal, 273
  Proctor's model of, 273

T

taxonomy, 185
teaching-learning process
  documenting, 169
  effectiveness, 170
  evaluation, 169
  steps, 167–170
teaching plan, 168–169
telehealth, 153–155, 300–301
  advantages, 153
  uses, 153
telemedicine
  consent form for, 154
  guidelines for, 154
  issues with, 154–155
  worldwide impact of, 154
theory of goal attainment, 42–43
theory of nursing systems, 44
theory of self-care, 44
Tompkins, Sally Louisa, 9–10
tort, 112
transcultural nursing, 48–49
Tripler Army Hospital, 12

U

unitary human being, 40
upward communication, 226
U.S. Public Health Service, 11

V

values, 92
veracity, 93
verbal communication, 226–228
  effective and ineffective, 228
Vietnam-era nurses, 13–14
village healer, 2
vulnerable populations, 135–138
  strategies to tackle health problems in, 137

W

WAVES (Women Accepted for Volunteer Emergency Service), 12
widows, 4
Women's Naval Reserve Act, 12
workplace incivility, 342
workplace violence, 341–342
  preventing, 342–344

Z

Zakrzewska, Marie, 10

www.ingramcontent.com/pod-product-compliance
Ingram Content Group UK Ltd.
Pitfield, Milton Keynes, MK11 3LW, UK
UKHW050141280726
14058UKWH00006B/773

9 781793 574305